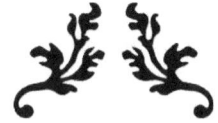

THE ECG MADE ABC

Let's keep the ECG Easy

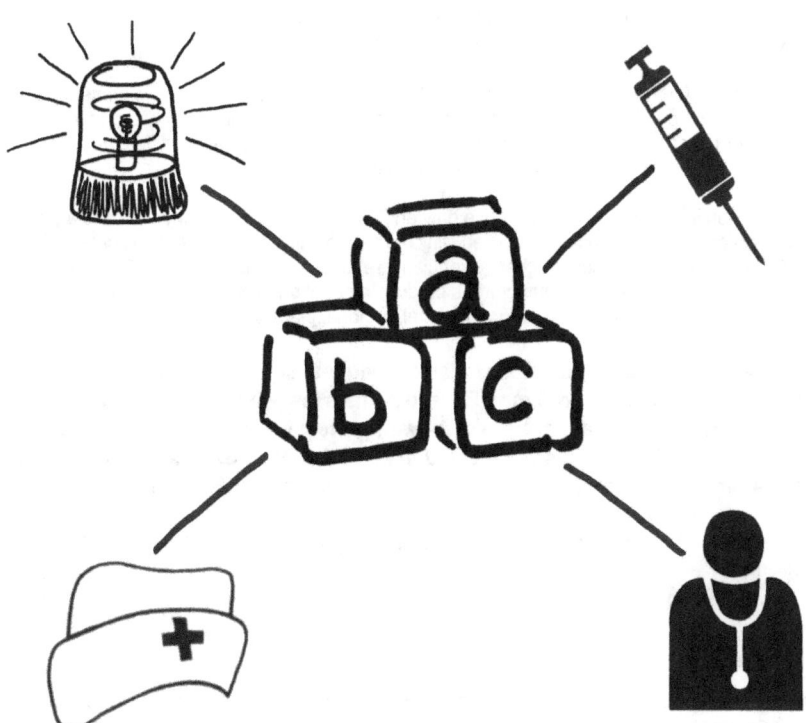

A Word Of Thanks

Just a few words I think to thank you to all those who helped me throw this new version together. A massive thanks to Declan, who has been a valued personal proof-reader and who offered advice (always constructive I have to say) where necessary.
To Nicky and Lou who have always encouraged me to get this sorted. To Kerrie for proof reading and correcting some of my grammar.
To everyone (way too many of you to mention) that have been asking for the new book and believed in me when there were times that I didn't believe in myself. Your demand for learning about ECGs is what keeps me going.
To Burt Manning one of the best instructors I know who taught me a lot about the basic way of teaching and learning, so if you don't like this book you can blame him as well! No seriously thanks, Burt I learned a lot from you. To Chris for putting up with all of this when it was a never ending "just doing a bit more on my book", you have had some patience with me thank you.
Finally, to Veronica at Burton Queens Hospital in Staffordshire, without you this project would never have got off the ground way back in 1997.

The biggest thank you goes to you, the reader. You have parted with your hard earned money to buy this and for that I will always be eternally grateful to you.

I hope you enjoy reading this book as much as I have enjoyed writing it. It took a long time to get together but I have also learnt a lot myself as a result.

If you have any comments, recommendations or suggestions, please let me know as they can only make this better. Please email me at theECGmadeABC@hotmail.com

Although every effort has been made to ensure that the information in this book is presently accurate, the author and the publishers do not accept responsibility or legal liability for any errors in the text or the misuse or misapplication of material in this work. If you notice any inaccuracies, errors or omissions, then please let me know using the above email.

The information in this book is for reference only and must not be used for any clinical diagnosis or clinical decisions. Please consult a qualified clinician before using any information contained in this book. As information and research change regularly, readers must ensure that they check with the most up to date and accurate manufacturer's product information, user manuals and any clinical procedures, guidelines and protocols for your local, regional, national health or private organisations.

This book is dedicated to all of our fallen colleagues, some taken way too soon. To Steve Wegg, Sam Orme and Simon Bear to name a few who have made a personal difference to me and others around them with professionalism, friendship and compassion. This book is also dedicated to all of the fallen ex or serving colleagues in whatever ambulance service or other health and medical profession.

The ECG Made ABC (previously known as Let's Make The ECG Easier To Understand © 2002) 1st Edition 2017

The ECG Made ABC

©2018 By Gareth J Mallon

Welcome to the fascinating world of the electrocardiograph or ECG. A subject much feared by many a medical student, nurse or ambulance person because "It is like learning a foreign language", partly to which I agree. The world of cardiology is very complex and like any language but it depends on how fluent you want to be. They are however easier to understand than you think when you understand the basics. Cardiologists are fluent at this language and specialists in their field but they also have spent many years specifically on this particular subject seeing countless ECGs and analysing them on a daily basis and even they are learning every day so we are not expected to be cardiologists, just able to speak in "pidgin". But who knows where this road may take you!

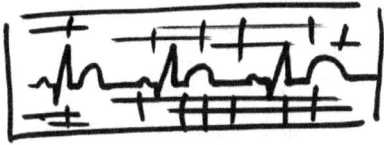

The first hurdle is that most medical books assume that you already have a high level of medical knowledge even before you open the front cover which can be very daunting and makes the going tough. It will make you less likely to want to learn about the subject before you even start. Many moons ago I was sent on an ECG recognition course which to be honest scared me witless (or another word that sounds the same!), as I knew absolutely nothing about ECGs except from television or in films where everyone ends up with a "flatline" on their monitor, they get successfully defibrillated (wrong!), survive without any side effects and the whole scene gets subjected to lots of dramatic music! Fortunately, on my course, I had a good teacher. He taught me on a level that even I could understand – A is for Apple, B is for Ball, and hopefully, I have passed on this way of teaching. If you want all the technical bits, there are plenty of good books out there to do that, if you want it basic then try this. Most books assume that you have a prior knowledge of some medical terminology and workings but not me. So I hope this book will help you to learn how to recognise the most common rhythms seen on the heart monitor that you may come across, by first explaining what is normal before we can work out what is not. However, also telling you why these things are happening and what to look for. It is not intended to blind you with technical stuff or give any in-depth treatments for the rhythms, just the bog standard basic way (and fun way I hope) of learning and understanding ECGs.

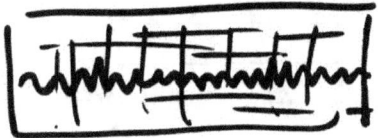

I want you to enjoy this book and not see it as just another chore, so I have tried to keep it as visual and as light-hearted as possible and to pass on the easiest way I know, to learn the basic way. The ECG is not too difficult to understand if you keep it simple, going into too much detail only fuzzes up the wrong brain cells. To be honest, the best way to tackle ECGs is to remember a few rules –

- Practise with as many ECG strips as you can get your hands on.
- Ask as many good doctors, nurses and specialists that you can find. Most will be happy to explain things to you.
- Don't look for something that is not there, if it shows a normal rhythm then it **is** usually a normal rhythm, look too hard and you will only confuse yourself. Just remember that there is a commonly used rule used in many a training room. The rule of K.I.S.S. - **K**eep **I**t **S**imple **S**tupid.
- Don't be afraid to have a guess and if you are really not sure, ask someone, nobody gets it right every time.

This book is designed for you to learn at your own pace so please feel free to jot down any notes on the pages if it helps. There is a blank notes page on 109 as well.

CONTENTS

I Didn't Know That!

I have read a few ECG books in my time but for whatever reason I had always wondered, really what is an ECG and where did it come from and when did it all begin, but no one ever seems to tell you. So I thought you might like a little insight into its origins. This is not a need to know, just a nice to know. So if you want to, just skip this bit. For those still reading here goes -

Believe it or not, a couple of British physiologists John Burden Sanderson and Frederick Page recorded the electrical current from of all things, a frog's heart using a capillary electrometer way back in 1887. It is believed that another British physiologist by the name of Augustus D. Waller published the first recorded ECG in1887.

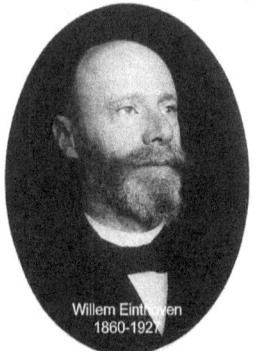

Willem Einthoven
1860-1927

Initially, he was convinced that this sort of thing could not be put to any use by anyone in the medical field, how wrong could he be? One of his colleagues, a Dutchman Willem Einthoven thought twice about this and decided to develop it further. He could see a difference in the ECG taken from a healthy person and one from a sick person and thought it could be of more benefit than first imagined.

Einthoven thought that he could improve on the simple capillary electrometer that was designed in 1887 by Clement Ader a French electrical engineer which was used by Waller at the time, so he set to work and modified and developed the string galvanometer, which although weighing 600 pounds did the job very well. He also suggested labelling the ECG splitting the rhythm into four sections and using the terminology P, QRS, T and U (why not ABC I cannot answer), which has remained universally unchanged to this day.

The result was an impressive quality ECG, but the biggest problem he had was that this monstrosity of an ECG machine weighed more than a quarter of a ton and it required no less than five people to operate it, a far cry from the portable systems of today!

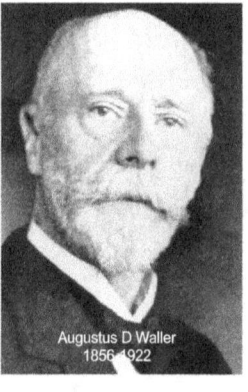

Augustus D Waller
1856-1922

The first commercial ECG machine available was in England in 1908 by the Cambridge Scientific Company and the first one sold for clinical use was by the University of Edinburgh. Just a year later the first hospitals to use it were the Sir Thomas Lewis at University College Hospital, London and the Mt Sinai Hospital, New York.

Such was the success of this venture that Einthoven and Lewis both strode ahead to improve what was a good thing. They had a series of meetings in the early 1900s and together developed the groundwork for what seemed like a remarkable discovery. This led to Einthoven being awarded the Nobel Prize for physiology and medicine in 1924. In 1928, things began to get a lot more portable. A company which was later to become Hewlett Packard condensed their static version into a 50-pound portable ECG machine powered by a 6-volt car battery.

They continued to pioneer this work until in the early 1930s, when Frank N. Wilson, who at this time was the most productive worker in the research into ECGs, concentrated his efforts on the QRS complex and T wave within the rhythm. He developed the unipolar (single direction) recording system by putting three electrodes placed on the left arm, the right arm and the left leg he could look at the hearts conduction from three different angles and effectively taking three different "pictures" of the heart. This became known as Einthoven's triangle (not to be confused with the Bermuda triangle!).

Development and studies of the ECG are widely researched and discussed throughout the world today and new discoveries are being made like the Brugada Syndrome in the 1980's and the new genetic link to cardiomyopathies, but the concept of the ECG and its terminology has remained unchanged since its birth and it is a universally recognised language. Isn't it amazing that we still use these basic principles for reading ECGs founded over a hundred years ago?

To this day the 12 lead ECG, which incidentally was pioneered in 1942, is able to take a more detailed picture of your heart and is a vital part of any clinical cardiology assessment (checking your ticker out). Did Waller realise that what he thought was a useless invention could produce well over 100 million ECG recordings worldwide every single year, I doubt it!

ECG Recorders

Historically, there were two ways in which ECG rhythms can be recorded; one of the older less used ways is by photographic methods using a beam of light, a mirror, a magnetic coil and some photographic paper. The mirror was mounted on a magnetic coil, which reflected the beam of light back and forth across the moving photo paper. The biggest drawback was the photo paper needed developing before the rhythm could be seen so you couldn't keep an eye on any changes happening.

This led to the development of pen recorders. Again these come in various sizes and guises.

The pen recorders physically write on moving paper so you have an instantaneous record as things are happening (or a hard paper copy as it is usually called) and are useful for diagnosing at any time or for filing away into a patient's records, or even as in our case, for learning purposes.

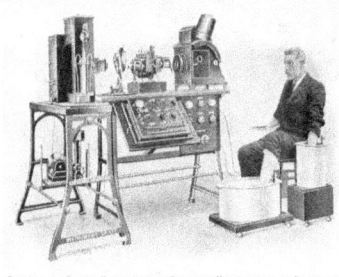

There are a couple of types of pen recorder. There is an ink filled version, this involves a thin tubed pen with an inkwell at one end and the other end it is connected to an electromagnet, which can move back and forth pretty fast. As the paper comes sideways out of the machine, the pen moves up and down the paper marking the paper as it comes out.

Another type that is more common is similar to above but there is no ink involved. Instead, an electrical current heats the tip and this marks the rhythm over the thermal paper (similar to fax machine paper, the paper turns black when heated). Even more modern again is a thin electrical strip, which is in contact with the ECG paper. This strip lays across the width of the paper and heated at various points along its path to produce the ECG, the advantage being is that it can cover a wide strip (usually about the A4 paper size) which means you could have lots of rhythms on one single ECG strip taken from different directions of the heart. Each lead is called a channel and the more channels the machine can print the more can be viewed on the single sheet of paper. So if an ECG machine is a single channel, then only one rhythm lead can be printed at any time. Consequently, a three channel machine can print 3 rhythm leads and so forth up to the 12 channel ECG machine which displays all 12 rhythm leads simultaneously. Also, there are no moving parts and is less likely to go wrong (so they say!)

These are the types of ways that you can record the ECG rhythm, but what if you only just want to monitor the patient? Well, it would be pretty silly to have reams of paper flowing out of a machine for 3 or 4 hours just in case you might see something because you will probably spend more time looking through it all and then never see anything anyway! Constant monitoring machines are usually the Holter-type monitor which the patient wears for between 24 hours and up to 7 days. These record real-time heart rhythms but usually have event markers to highlight any abnormalities. This is usually either the machine's software analysis or by the wearer pressing an "event" button on the monitor when they feel unwell or get any palpitations or heart irregularities.

There are some types of displays available; the older machines used to be the oscilloscope. This type of machine is used by many an electrical engineer, gives an excellent quality display and is capable of recording low voltages. This is an ideal choice of display but they are not cheap, so the other type, which is becoming the more affordable option, is the Liquid Crystal Display (LCD) screen. These are similar to the sort of screens you would find on basic and older mobile phones and some games consoles. While they do not cost as much as

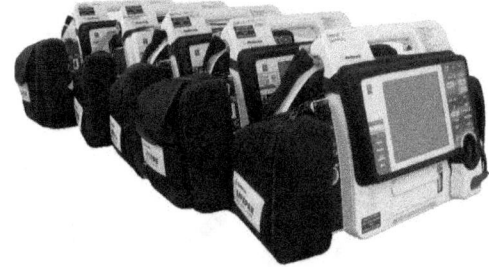

an oscilloscope, most of the modern ECG monitors are also multi-function devices incorporating other forms of monitoring such as pulse oximetry, capnography, and blood pressure monitors so are a better form of the multi-monitoring device.

Technology has advanced immensely over the years from Einthoven's quarter ton monster to the modern machines, which are even down to something the size of a small pencil case that fit between your fingers and on the end of a stethoscope! Most machines are now so advanced that they are able with the use of some clever diagnostic software to diagnose an ECG helping us, but they are just a computer and work on a set of strict algorithms and parameter so the only way for definitive diagnosis is a human. Another excellent capability of technology is telemetry or Bluetooth and, of course, the internet with the ability to send ECG readings directly from the monitor and down the telephone line or over the web instantly to a person who could be hundreds or even thousands of miles away. So a patient's personal physician in America could diagnose a person on holiday in England while they are still wired up to the monitor!

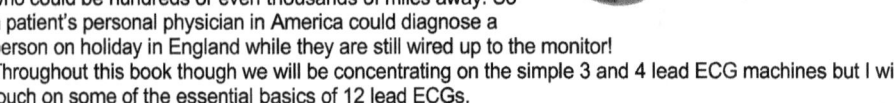

Throughout this book though we will be concentrating on the simple 3 and 4 lead ECG machines but I will touch on some of the essential basics of 12 lead ECGs.

With A Little Help From My Friends

To help things along and to make things a little lighter hearted, I have recruited a few friends; I hope they make life a bit easier.

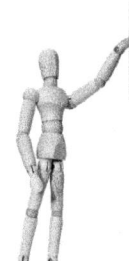

Here is something that we are talking about at the time.

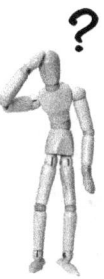

If you see this little friend who looks a little confused, advising you that this might be something tricky or a bit technical and you might have to put the old grey matter to the test. So take your time and you'll get there.

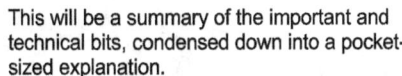

This will be a summary of the important and technical bits, condensed down into a pocket-sized explanation.

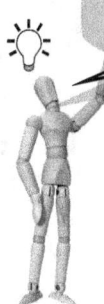

Welcome To The Learning Zone

It is time now to get out your thinking cap and put the old grey matter to use.
Please take your time, and go through each section in turn.
Remember, though; I <u>will</u> be asking questions later.
Just don't forget, it is as simple as ABC. It will
A ll
B ecome
C lear

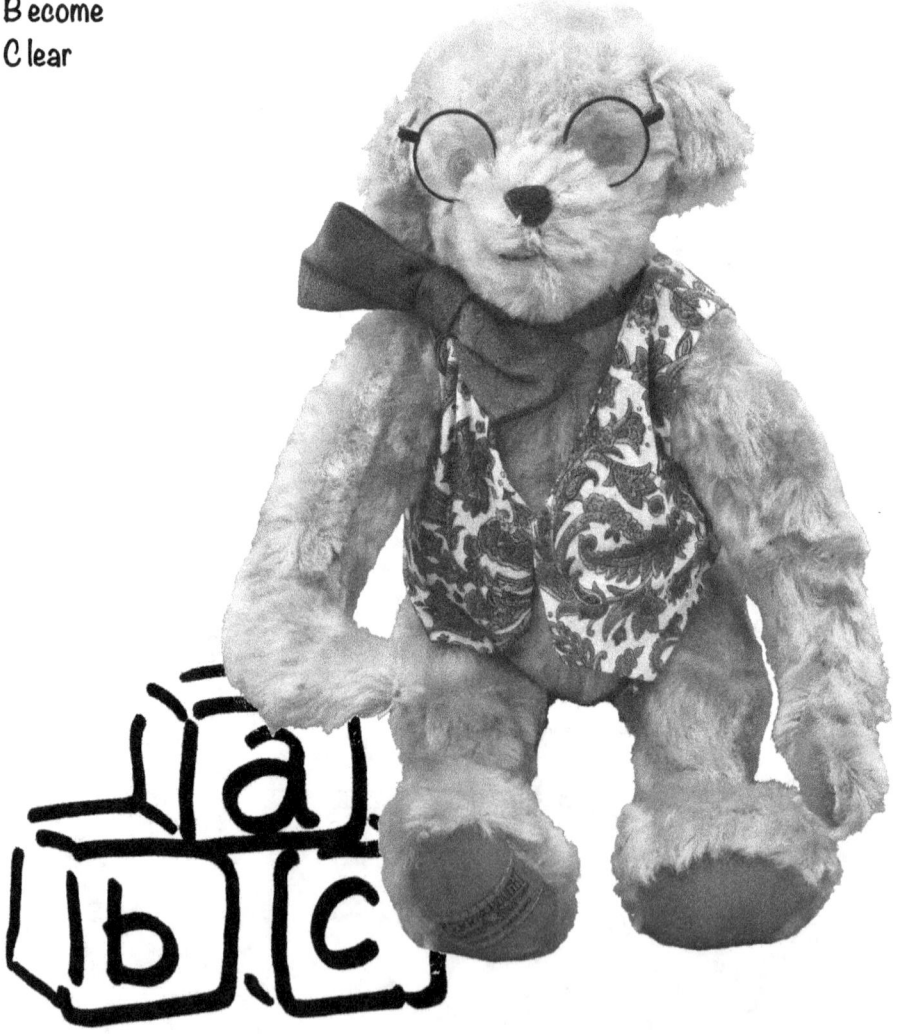

The Heart, What is it?

You should be able to recognise the basic ECG heart rhythm within 45 seconds. Some can take just a bit longer; others may take only a few seconds (we call these the Oh dear! rhythms which will be explained later). The best way to start this is to learn the basics about the activity of the heart both mechanically and electrically, so please bear with me if we follow over old ground.

Isn't nature an amazing creature? To think that since the dawn of time (well, Adam and Eve times anyway!), there has never been a Mark 2 human. Things like cars and computers are upgraded with the latest software or engine and suspension design but the human never has. There were no doctors or nurses in caveman times, so nature would provide its own way coping or warning you that it was not functioning well and needed attention.

The heart as we know is the most efficient mechanical pump known to us. It has never been synthetically replicated (copied to you and me!) to last as long or to work as efficiently as nature's version since time began. True, surgeons have implanted many a mechanical heart saving many lives, but they have yet to design something that is as effective in its long term low maintenance and robust construction such is the human heart which has so many fail-safe devices built in. It is capable of working 24 hours a day 365 days a year and if we are fortunate, quite efficiently for up to and over 100 years. In its lifetime, it will beat approximately 2.5 billion times and that is some achievement. It can regulate its self and to make small repairs if damaged for example by rerouting some of the coronary arteries (depending on the damage). It is ultimately the body's engine and it will do all it can to keep it running even though it may misfire as without it none of our other organs would survive. If you would like to know approximately how much blood that the heart would pump around in its lifetime, you would have to open your kitchen tap fully for approx. 45 years. Now that is some going!

Also how amazing is nature to put your heart (the most important organ for survival) between an armoured bone (sternum), surrounded by a flexible cage (ribs) and a rigid pole behind (spine) so that in the event that the heart stopped working, you could press the plate (chest compressions) onto the rigid pole and with the flexibility of the cage, the correct depth of compression and the correct rate, you could even kick start the heart to pump again by doing good CPR. How cool is nature that after millions of years we have only just worked this one out!

As for its construction, it is a hollow muscular organ, about the size of the owner's fist in an adult and is located behind the sternum. It is actually upside down (the top or apex is at the bottom and the base is at the top). This is because we are born our heart it forms into four chambers, closes up and rotates as it develops in the womb.

The heart I suppose it could be compared to, say a washing machine or car petrol pump. It works both mechanically and electrically and one can't function without the other, if there is a fault in either of them, then the other becomes affected. The heart works on the same principle; then this means the motor could misfire and not run smoothly, consequently if the engine is damaged (i.e. heart attack) then the wiring could be put under strain.

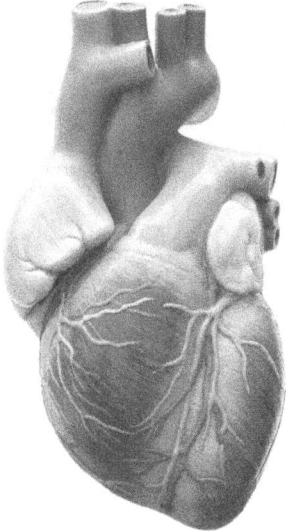

Have A Heart

As we mentioned on the previous page, the heart works both mechanically and electrically. So let's have a look at a cutaway view of the heart and see where the two separate internally so to speak.

To help you with this, all the electrical components have this spark plug symbol next to them and the others are the mechanical or structural ones.

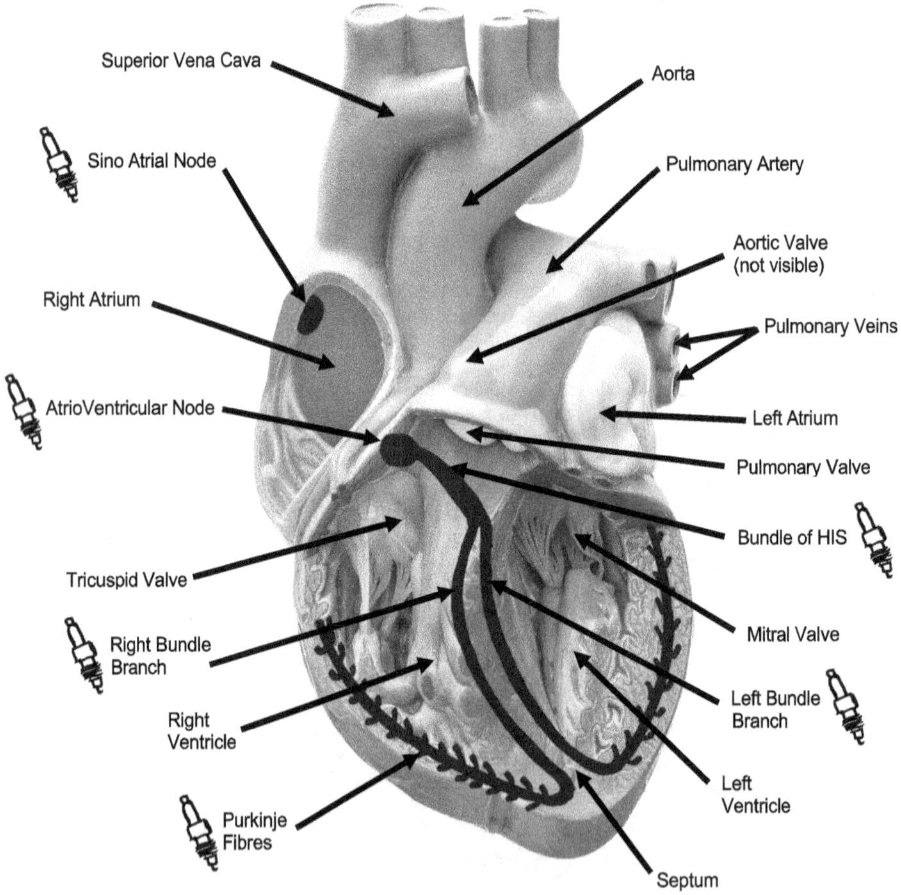

Superior Vena Cava

Sino Atrial Node

Right Atrium

AtrioVentricular Node

Tricuspid Valve

Right Bundle Branch

Right Ventricle

Purkinje Fibres

Aorta

Pulmonary Artery

Aortic Valve (not visible)

Pulmonary Veins

Left Atrium

Pulmonary Valve

Bundle of HIS

Mitral Valve

Left Bundle Branch

Left Ventricle

Septum

Let's Go Down To, Electric Avenue

? We talk about the electrical function of the heart but how does it make the electricity? Well, it's all due to alchemy. Just like the old days when we had chemistry and science sets for Christmas and created more than just electricity!

Let's go back to basics again for something that is of relevance to some of the fast heart rates (tachycardias) later in the book.

The sodium-potassium pump is most peoples' nightmare. So, what is it all about then and what is an action potential? Well, electrical impulse comes from something called ions. These are electrically charged particles which are formed when atoms lose or gain electrons (electrons are the negatively charged particles of an atom).

Woah!! For goodness sake lets slow down and take a breath, this is getting too complicated! Ok, keeping it basic, electricity is made by the sodium-potassium (also with the help of calcium) ions moving in and out of the semi-permeable (a bit like a cheese cloth) cell membrane and move between the intracellular and extracellular (inside and outside the cell) and moving between a low gradient to a high gradient to equal each other out. As three potassium ions move into the cell and two sodium move out (with the help of a protein called ATPase or Angiotensin) it creates a positive charge. The action potential is a sort of explosion of activity.

The way that the cells work is that when a cell discharges following immediately behind is the "refractory" and repolarising (recharging or numb) phase where any stimulus would make no difference and would still stay numb. The diagram below shows a very simple explanation of an action potential.

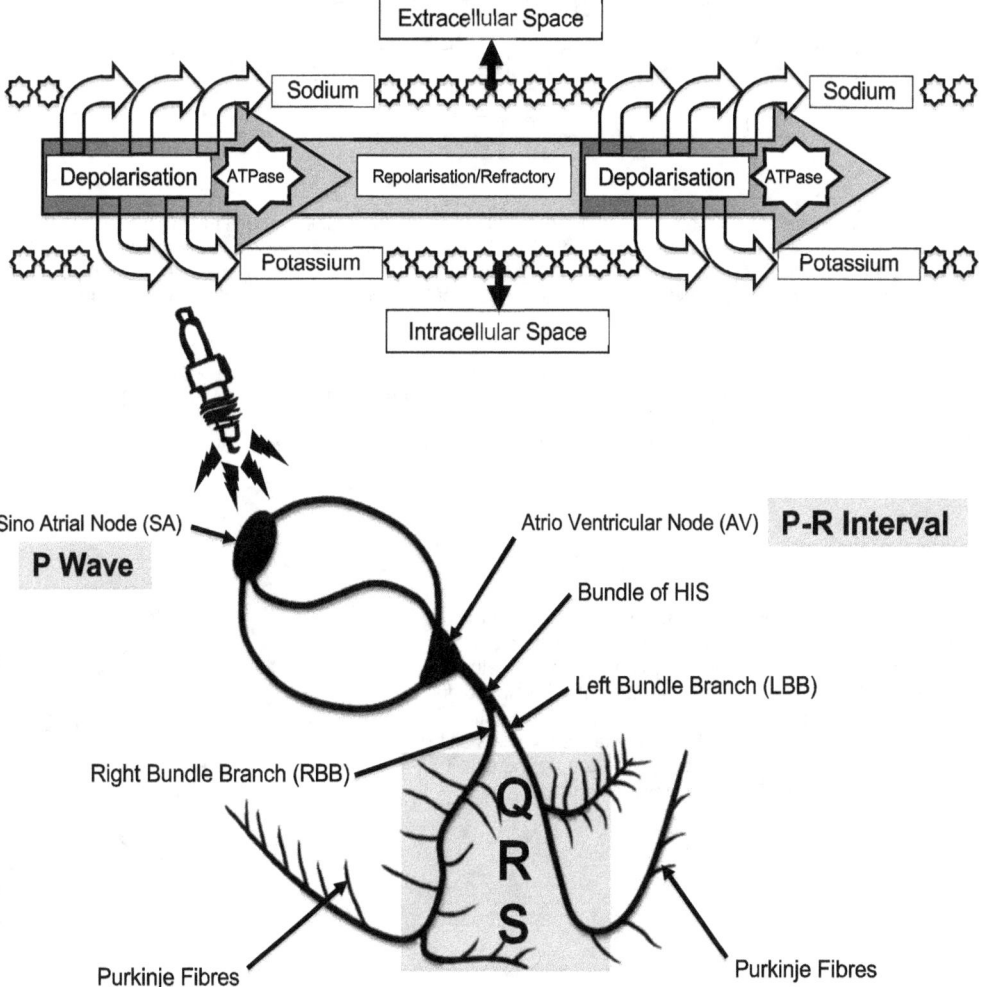

This is all good and well when things go well but continuing the common theme of the ECG and, of course, this book, sometimes things go wrong and if they do then we need to know why.

As we discussed, the cell produces an action potential and that is followed by a refractory period as it recharges. Sometimes individual cells do not understand the rule and they play their own game. This could be because they are diseased or just because they can, and why not???

Re-entry is the mechanism (capable of producing or promoting an arrhythmia) by which a wave of excitation turns upon itself and then re-enters the tissue that had been previously activated.

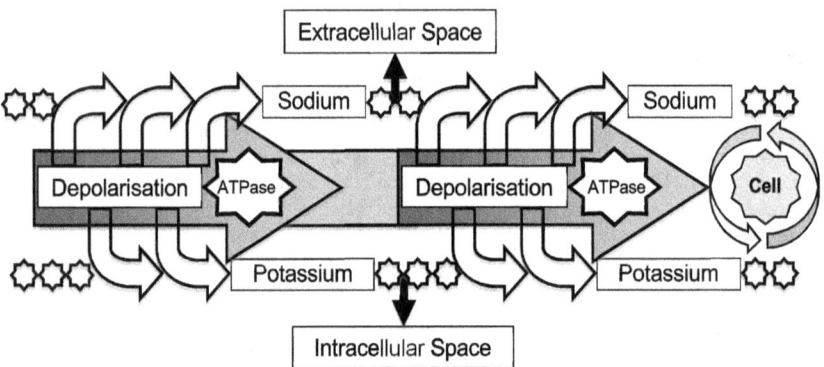

What normally happens with the cardiac impulse is that it would move rapidly through the heart and then it would extinguish as it makes its pass through the heart following with refractory period (the amount of time it takes for the excitable membrane to be ready to fire again). This means that the impulse has nowhere to go. Under the right conditions, it could be possible for any part of the myocardium or conduction system to support re-entry circuit

There are a number of reasons and many forms and causes for arrhythmias but as this is a basic book (ABC), we will concentrate on the simple re-entry aspect of this. When you see this symbol, it lets you know that this is caused by re-entry foci.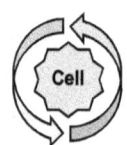

Some cells (usually adjacent to each other) have no refractory period and are constantly excitable so are vulnerable to any stimulus. So guess what happens, yup, they are prematurely activated. This will cause them to permanently fire off and get caught in a vicious re-entry cycle which will continue until terminated by drugs, defibrillation or worse, death. It is a bit like a dog chasing its tail. Until you stop it, it will keep going until it becomes exhausted and will stop (cardiac arrest).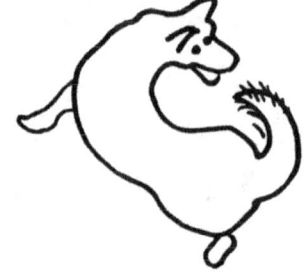

Let's Get Down To Basics

As we mentioned earlier in the book, the basic heart construction consists of four chambers. The top two are the atria (receiving chambers) and the lower two are called the ventricles (pumping chambers). The atrial chambers are separated and sealed from the ventricles by one-way valves to prevent any blood flowing back while lying down or doing handstands and things! The atria are separated from the ventricles by a nonconductive muscle so the electrical activity has to follow the determined pathway through the correct wiring but the internal surfaces are still conductive.

All four are divided down the middle by something called the septum, thus giving us our four chambers. The right side of the heart deals with receiving deoxygenated blood from the body (**R**ight-**R**ubbish) in the right atria, and also for pumping blood to then to the lungs via the right ventricle. The left side deals with receiving oxygenated blood from the lungs into the left atria, and the left ventricle pumps blood to the body's organs and systems.

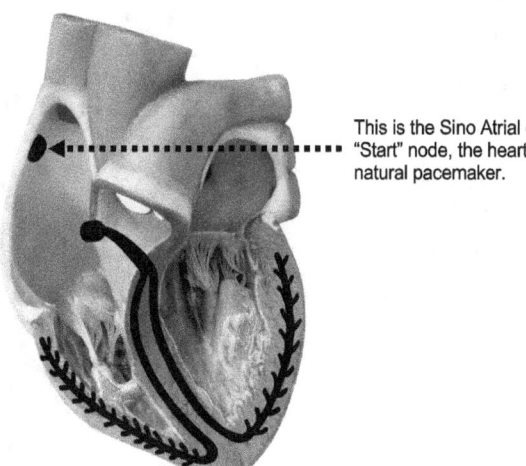

Right Atrium / Left Atrium (Receiving chambers)

One-way valve

Septum

Right Ventricle / Left Ventricle (Pumping chambers)

Because of the high pressure needed to pump the blood throughout the whole body the, walls of the left ventricle are much thicker and have a greater contractual force than the right side.

To make the blood pump, the atria and the ventricles have to contract to squeeze the blood to the lungs and the organs. This is done by a chemical reaction of sodium, potassium and calcium (know strangely as the sodium-potassium pump). The squeeze is the electrical action called "depolarisation". When the muscle rests, it is known as "repolarisation". These changes are detected and recorded by an ECG monitor.

The electrical discharge is a controlled electrocution (effectively "tasering the muscle) to make them tense, hence, squeeze the chambers creating the pumping action

The electrical impulses have a predetermined pathway to follow, which starts in the right atrium and is called the sinoatrial (**SA**) node (or the "S"t"A"rt node). This is the heart's natural pacemaker and like all cardiac nodes is made up of a mass of specialised nerve cells embedded high up into the heart wall in the right atria. It has its own blood supply from the Right Coronary Artery (RCA) and under

This is the Sino Atrial or "Start" node, the heart's natural pacemaker.

normal circumstances will fire at about 60 to 100 Beats Per Minute (BPM) controlled by nerves, but it can only handle a maximum speed of a about 140 BPM before it gives up and the cells in the atria take over (see next).

Within the walls of the atria are millions of excitable and conductive cells each one capable of firing on its own accord, or when linked together spread to the next cell then to the next and so on down the line. They are specialised cardiac cells only found in the heart. When the impulse leaves the SA node (moving from superior (top) to inferior (bottom) and right to left, it excites the nearest cell which in turn excites the next one to it and so on creating something very similar to a Mexican wave throughout the atria. This simultaneously contracts the two atria shortening the sheet of atrial muscle, pumping blood through the one-way valves down to the ventricles. The impulse stops at this point and does not go automatically to the ventricles as this would just make the heart explode! The electricity is blocked by a sheet of nonconductive muscle separating the atria from the ventricles. Because the right atrium contracts slightly before the left, it pumps in a slightly clockwise twisting motion.

Only 30% of the blood is pumped to the ventricles; the remaining 70% is passed down by gravity, which is important to remember in certain cardiac conditions and rhythms such as Atrial Fibrillation (see page 51).

When the atrial impulse reaches its end it is picked up by the AtrioVentricular (**AV**) node or the "A"rf "V"ay (Half Way node). This node is like a relay and holding station and holds on to this impulse for a brief moment before passing it down the **Bundle of HIS** and to the ventricles. If there is a hole (commonly known as an accessory pathway) in the muscle separating the atria from the ventricles, the impulse could "leak" through and pre-excite (prematurely contract) the ventricles before their correct turn and this could cause the heart to go into some serious (Supra Ventricular

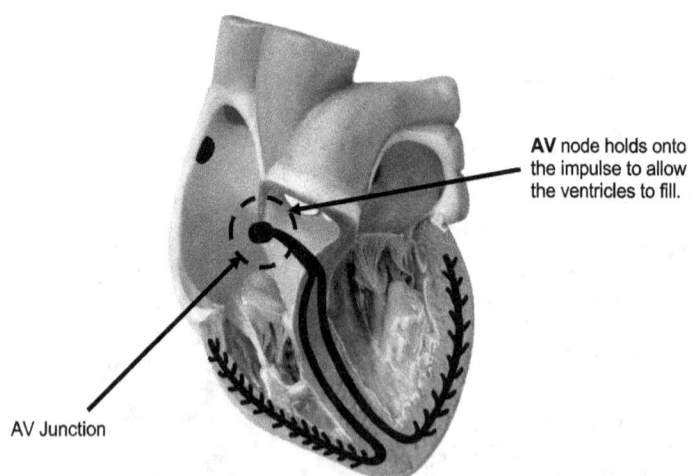

AV node holds onto the impulse to allow the ventricles to fill.

AV Junction

Tachycardia) or life-threatening rhythms such as Ventricular Tachycardia (see page 73). The most common rhythm for this is an inherited condition called Wolfe Parkinson White Syndrome (WPW).

The AV node also has a safety device to protect the ventricles from rapid impulses such as Atrial Fibrillation (AF).

The ventricular impulse first passes down the **Bundle of HIS** (named after a German doctor who discovered it called Mr HIS), which looks like an upturned tuning fork and called the **bundle branches**. The impulse starts in the left branch side, and then travels over to the right (this is important to remember to determine if a heart block could be left or right). The left bundle branch feeds the left ventricles and the right branch supplies the right. They both travel down and around and down to the bottom of the heart (or the apex) to the spidery type nerves embedded in the ventricular walls known as **Purkinje fibres**. As with the atria, these then excite the cells in the muscle and cause them to contract and shorten both ventricles simultaneously, pumping the blood again through one-way valves around the body through the arteries. Again, because of the small delayed impulse from the left to the right ventricle it pumps in a slightly clockwise twisting motion.

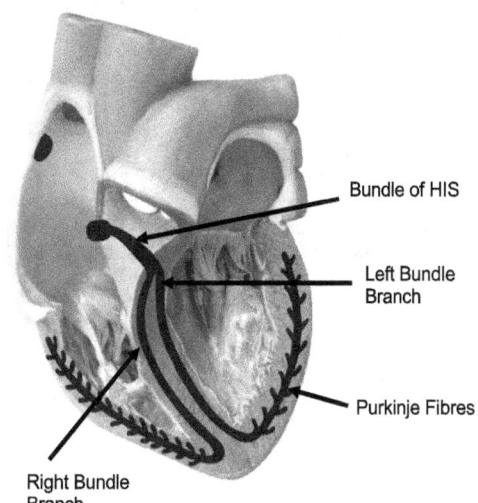

Bundle of HIS

Left Bundle Branch

Purkinje Fibres

Right Bundle Branch

To Sum It All Up

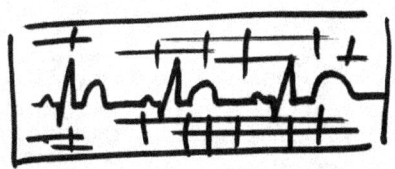

So the electrical path followed from start to finish would be,

- **SA** node (the pacemaker).
- Controlled tasering and Mexican wave across the atria (simultaneous contraction and shortening of both atria).
- **AV** node
- A short delay (to allow the ventricles to fill).
- Down the **bundle of HIS.**
- Left and right **bundle branches** (Upside down tuning fork), first from the left side then to the right side.
- **Purkinje fibres.**
- Controlled tasering and Mexican wave across the ventricles (simultaneous contraction of both ventricles).

Let's Get Connected!

It is time to connect up our poor unsuspecting soul to the ECG monitor! Electrodes (or "dots" as they are often called) are used to transmit the electrical activity of the heart, from the skin's surface to an ECG monitor. But how do we do it and where do we connect the leads? Well, fortunately, a person who was mentioned earlier, a Mr Einthoven worked this one out for us and, strangely enough, he called it Einthoven's triangle.

It goes as follows - You will usually find three leads coming from the machine, labelled **RA** (Right Arm), **LA** (Left Arm) and **LL** (Left Leg). These might also be colour coded as **RA** (red), **LA** (yellow) and **LL** (green or black). Most commercial ECG machines now have **Four** leads just to confuse matters, if this is the case, connect up the three leads as shown (see diagram below), then place the fourth one on the right leg. If you are still not sure, you may have to consult the manufacturer's user manual for more details.

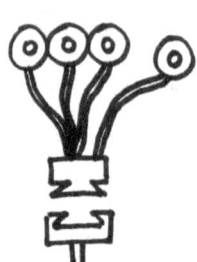

The leads are connected up using the electrodes to form a virtual triangle on the body. The most common place used to be on the shoulders and the abdomen but more recent guidelines are to place the leads on the end of the limbs on the wrists and ankles. This is especially important when adding the extra chest leads for 12 lead monitoring. If you are in doubt, then please consult your most recent training guidelines or contact your training department for advice.

A NOTE TO REMEMBER - Before you start wiring up anyone to the monitor, please remember to tell them what you are doing at all times as not to alarm or upset them; the idea of being wired to a heart monitor can conjure up all sorts of fears about what could be wrong or what might be found. Also, it will give you a better and more accurate reading, as hopefully they should be more relaxed.

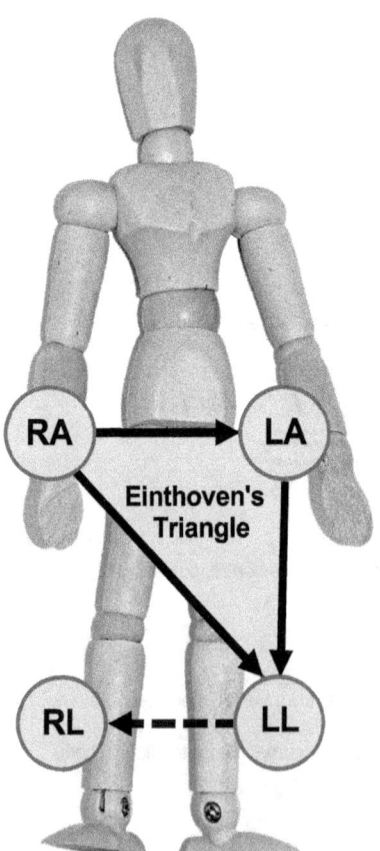

Einthoven's Triangle

- The **RA** lead (1) is placed on the **right wrist**
- The **LA** (2) on the **left wrist**
- The **LL (3)** placed on the **left leg.**

This should give us our Einthoven's triangle, now we can now look at the heart from three different directions.

Note: If you have four leads (which most commercial ECG machines have) place the last one (4) on the **right ankle.** You will find on your machine that there are three lead settings, **lead I, II and III** (these will view the heart from 3 different angles). We will concentrate on just these 3 lead settings from now on

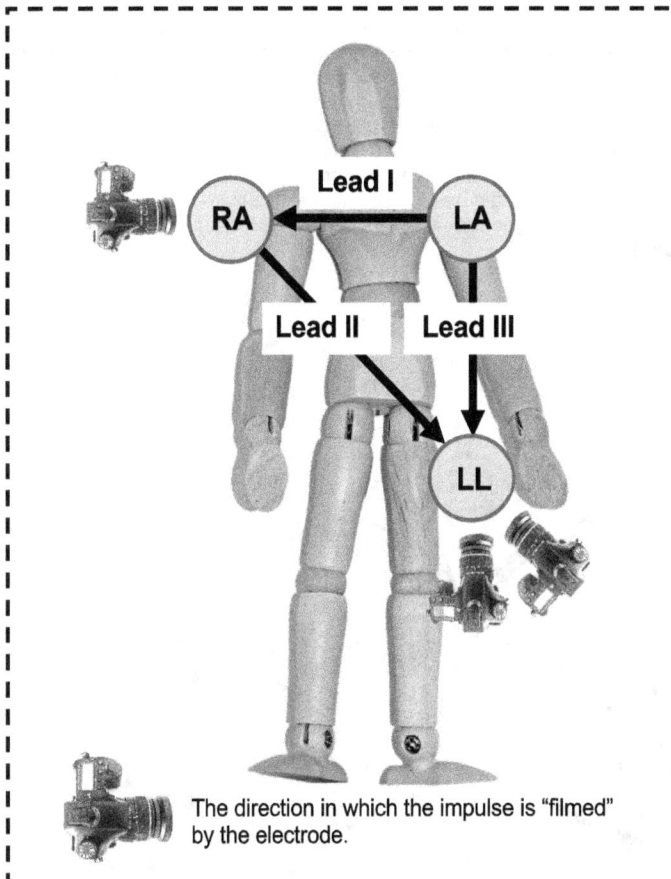

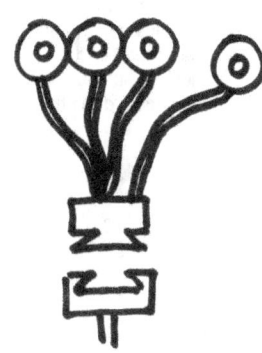

Lead I

Lead II   Lead III

RA   LA

LL

The direction in which the impulse is "filmed" by the electrode.

- **Lead I** will look at the heart from the **Left Arm (LA)** to the **Right Arm (RA)** lead (or L shoulder to the R shoulder).
- **Lead II** will look from the **RA** to the **Left Leg (LL)** lead. As this direction follows the heart's natural electrical pathway, then this is the most common one used for monitoring someone (R shoulder to the L abdomen).
- **Lead III** is from the **Left Arm** to the **Left Leg (LL)** lead (the L shoulder to the L abdomen).

RA Red

LA Yellow

LL Green/Black

RL The odd one out (Right Leg)

Think,
Ride
Your   Or Even
Green
Bike!

Traffic
Lights!
Red
Yellow
Green

And Now For Something A Bit Different

An interesting question that was mused over some time ago in the wee hours of a Sunday morning was, what if a person was buried up to their neck (feet first of course!) in something like a sand pit or tunnel cave-in or a similar accident, then where would you put the leads to monitor them? Well after many minutes of profound and meaningful discussions and many deep and strong cups of coffee it was thought the only way to find out is to have a go, so a cave in was simulated using two armchairs and a tea cosy (don't ask!) and it was found that in amongst the fits of laughter, spilt coffee and the occasional passing "what's the tea cosy for?" question, that it was actually possible to connect someone to an ECG monitor by wiring up their ears, nose or forehead to the machine as long as you get the LL lead (the green or black one) as far down the chest as you could reach. This created would you believe a perfectly normal looking ECG reading, but please kids, don't try this at home!

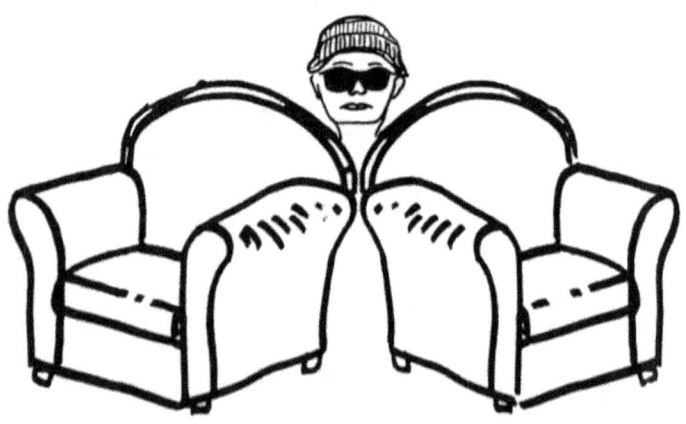

Let's Get 12 Leads From 10

As technology has now advanced considerably over the last few years, 12 lead diagnostic ECG machines have now become more common on the wards and departments and more common in A+E ambulances and GP surgeries so you are more likely to get the chance to use one of these.

The inclusion of this section is a nice to know because correct ECG diagnosis is only possible using 12 leads and this is becoming increasing common for all levels of medical staff to be able to perform this efficiently and accurately.

The correct placements of these leads are far more critical than the three or four lead ECG readings as the 12 lead reading takes an accurate reading of the heart, from all angles, left, right, up, down, top and bottom. With practice though you can put these on quite quickly and accurately. Before you dive into putting on these extra leads (they call it 12 leads but you only physically use 10 leads in total), connect up the normal chest and limb leads as described on page 17.

It is best to start with the V_1 lead. First, on the right hand side of the patient's chest find the Angle of Louis by sliding your fingers under both collar bones down to the notch just above the sternum (this is not easy to do, so you may have to practise to get the feel of this), then count another three rib spaces down then place the first electrode in this fourth intercostal space just to the right of the sternum. The V_2 lead then goes in the same intercostal space just to the left of the sternum. Place the V_4 lead next. Find the midway point between the clavicle that joins at the sternum and the shoulder, draw an imaginary line straight down the chest to the fifth intercostal space (just count down one more space from lead V_2). Place the V_3 lead between V_2 and V_4 on the 5th rib. V_5 goes in a horizontal line from V_4 in line with the shoulder and finally V_6 is placed again level with V_4 in a vertical line with the crease of the armpit. So –

- V_1 – In the **fourth** intercostal space to the right of the sternum
- V_2 – In the **fourth** intercostal space to the left of the sternum
- V_3 – On the **fifth** rib in between V_2 and V_4
- V_4 – In the **fifth** intercostal space in the mid clavicle line
- V_5 – **In line with V_4** and in a vertical line down from the shoulder
- V_6 – Again **in line with V_4** and in a vertical line down from the armpit crease

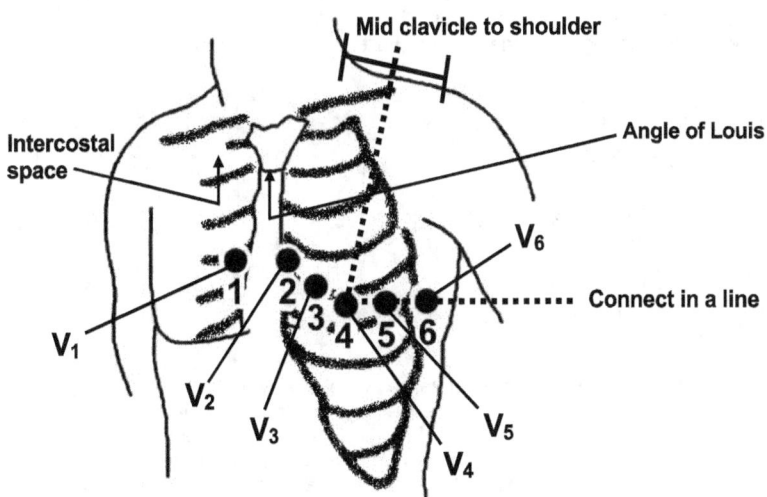

Don't Interfere Please

Quite often when monitoring someone, the quality of the ECG reading might not be very clear. The main reasons for this are usually poor or loose connections to the machine, the sticky electrodes have not stuck properly, or they may need moving to get a better reading. People with hairy chests may cause you a problem or two as the sticky electrodes no matter how sticky, do not stick very well to hair and as the electrodes need to be in direct contact with skin, the only way around this is to shave them and get down to skin, but having someone diving at your chest wielding a razor could be a bit alarming so please tell them what you are doing first! If all is well then check the connections of your leads and stickiness of the electrodes (as the gel can dry out sometimes). If they are ok, check your patient. See if they are moving around or shivering or they have difficulty breathing. Some people may have Parkinson's disease or Multiple Sclerosis (MS) and those who are hypothermic or agitated cannot control their shaking; all of these movements can cause interference to your reading. If so, try to relax them as much as possible. If you can't then try moving the electrodes to places that don't move as much, try the RA and LA, the tops of the arms, and maybe moving the LL lead to the left thigh or lower legs. This can sometimes solve your problem or may give you a clearer reading.

The rhythm below as an example is actually a normal rhythm but it has some muscle tremor, which could confuse you into thinking that it was a problem rhythm.

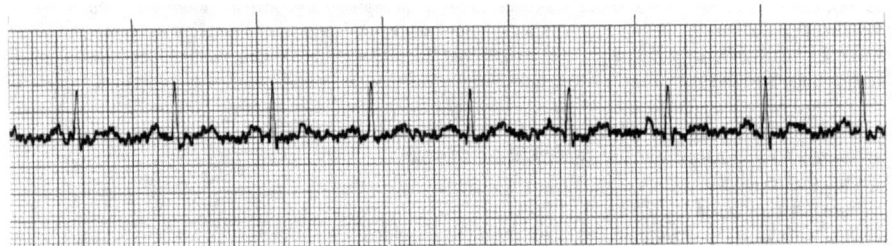

Another problem you may get is called the **"Wandering Baseline"**. When a patient has breathing difficulties then they tend to use their chest muscles a lot more to help them, this can cause the reading to look rather wavy. You will see the rhythm rise up over the baseline on breathing in and down on breathing out.
Below is an example of "Wandering Baseline" rhythm (for baseline see page 24) rhythm, which can be caused by the chest, leads moving on a person with breathing problems. If you suspect that someone's breathing might cause a poor reading, try connecting the chest leads and see if that helps.

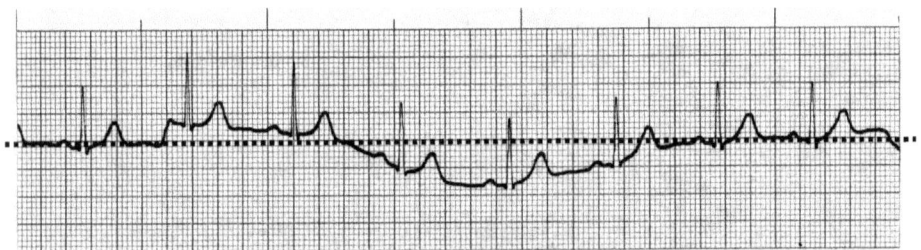

Sometimes overlooked is the possible cause of interference by electrical appliances like a syringe pump, mobile phone, fridge, television, table lamps (especially energy bulbs) or even an electric blanket. If you can, keep the person you are monitoring away from electrical things (not easy sometimes!), or try repositioning the electrodes or move the monitor further away from what you think is causing the interference. Also, remember that the type of person that you are monitoring can influence the type of signal you may see. For instance, when looking at an ECG from a large person you might see a small QRS complex due to the fact that the signal has to go through lots of fatty tissue before it is picked up on the body's surface. A person with emphysema will also give off a small QRS complex as the signal has to go through a lot of air pockets (due to the lung problem) before it reaches the surface.

The Paper Work

Seeing an ECG rhythm on a screen is ok if you are there to watch it all the time and have a photographic memory, but like the majority of us who can't, then the only answer is a hard copy printout for reference, analysis or for just putting into your pocket for a later date, then finding it after a 40-degree biological wash where everything, including the ECG strip, is now whiter than white! (Oh, by the way never try and laminate a thermal ECG printout, I found this out the hard way!).

What we can do is to link up this action to what comes up on the ECG screen, but first let's run through a bit about the ECG machine itself. There are loads of different makes and models on the market, so I won't be giving examples using on any particular type of monitor or recorder but they all give roughly the same results anyway and are fairly universal worldwide (see page 6).

To make life a bit easier all ECG machines use the same scale paper and all should kick this out at the same speed which is 25mm/sec, so no matter what machine you or anyone you know uses you can be safe that there shouldn't be too many differences in the reading of the rhythm (but if in doubt then read the user manual that comes with your machine). Which means if you can get someone to get hold of as many different types of rhythms strips as you can and practise, practise, practise!! There are many ECG websites and practice strips on the internet but be careful of sometimes conflicting information, and try and stick to reputable or government sites.

The electrical side of the heart gives off an electrical signal due to chemical changes and is picked up through the skin and recorded on an ECG monitor either as a positive (+) or as a negative (-) signal, if it goes up it's positive if it goes down it's negative, simple really. The monitor is similar to the types used by electrical engineers to test printed circuits and components so we are not talking high voltages here.

As for the ECG paper, it is of a simple grid type construction and is split into two types of squares, either small or large.

The paper comes out of the machine sideways, so along its length is recorded the time. Then up and down the paper records the voltage in millivolts.

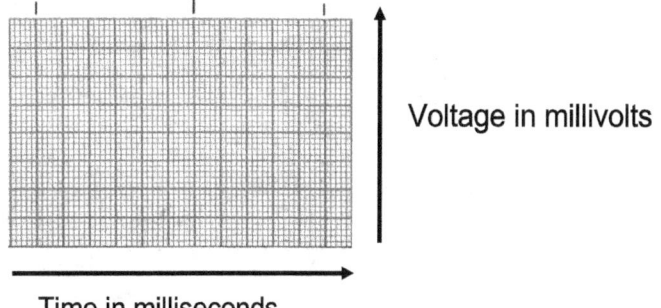

Voltage in millivolts

Time in milliseconds

Each small square on the paper is equivalent in time as 0.04 sec, and each large square (5 small squares) is equivalent to 0.2 sec. So 5 large squares would equal 1 second of time.

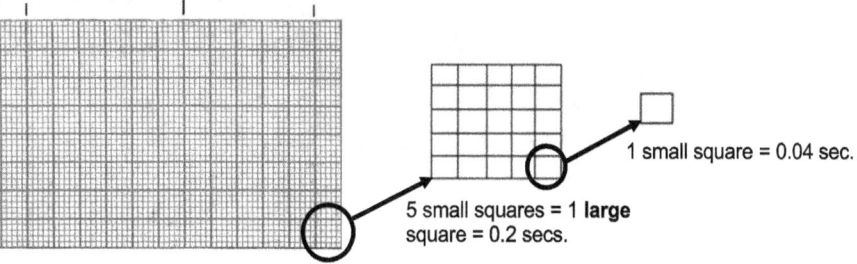

5 small squares = 1 **large** square = 0.2 secs.

1 small square = 0.04 sec.

Just The Right Calibre

A point worth noting and is often overlooked but is never the less quite important is the ability on most ECG machines to increase or decrease the size of the ECG rhythm for ease of clarity. For example, sometimes it may help to magnify the image twice or maybe four times its size to look closer at the P waves, or maybe the ECG voltages may be too small to read and need a bit of a boost. Or it could be that the ECG voltages are too big or there is a lot of interference and need reducing to try and smooth out the rhythm.

Default calibration setting. Note X1.0 setting is two large squares high. This is confirmed by the printed information shown below.

Normal ECG size of 1mv. This is the default setting.

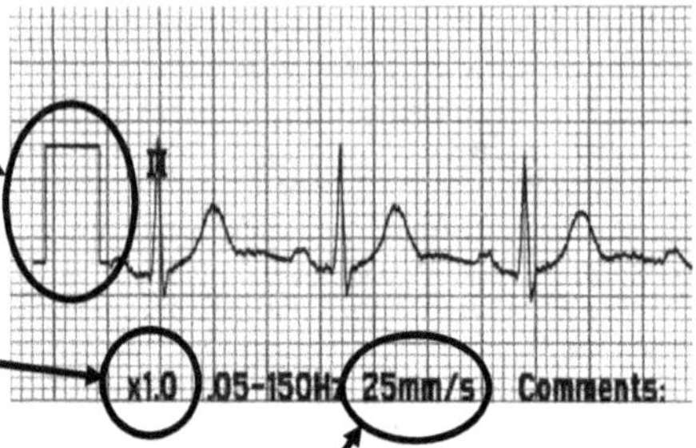

The default setting paper speed of 25mm per second.

Calibration setting. The larger size of X2.0 is 4 large squares high.

Twice the normal ECG size.

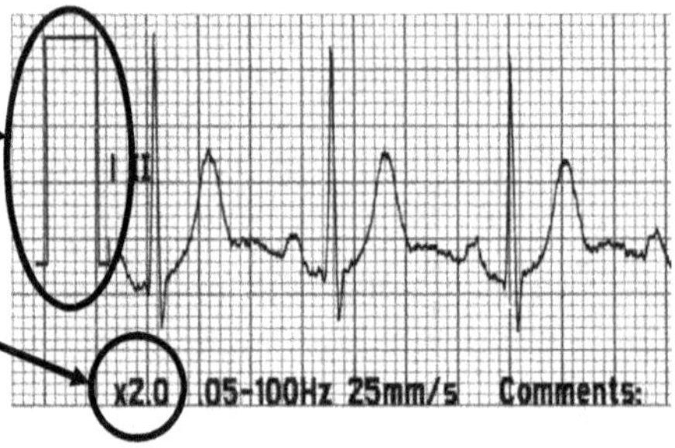

Calibration setting. ½ the size and is 1 large square high.

Half the normal ECG size.

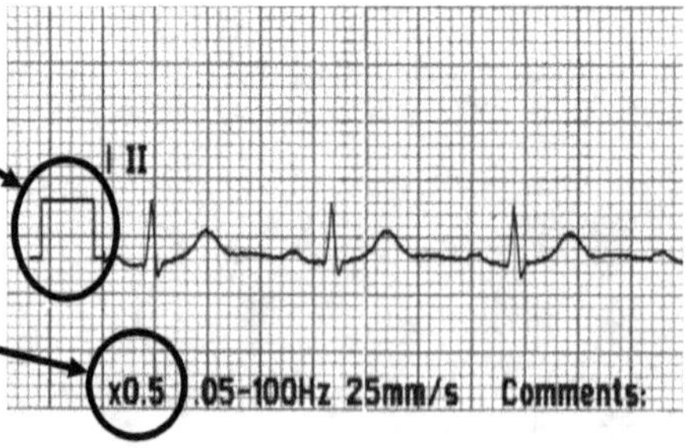

Well, before the ECG machine can give you a reading whether it is on the screen or printed, it needs to be calibrated. Without this, how would you know if the reading is accurate? The machine's usual default calibration setting is 1.0mv (two large squares) or X1.0. This is the standard setting that most ECG strips will be presented. This is usually automatically printed on many modern-day ECG machines and should show up on most ECG rhythm strips. There are though a few machines that do not print the calibration settings, ECG voltage size and the paper speed on the hard copy. If your machine is not capable of this, you must make a note on the presenting rhythm strip to avoid confusion or misdiagnosis, especially if you have altered the size of the ECG printout.

It's As Simple As ABC

The letters used in describing each ECG heartbeat are **P, PR Interval, QRS** and **T** in that order; each one represents a different part of the complex.

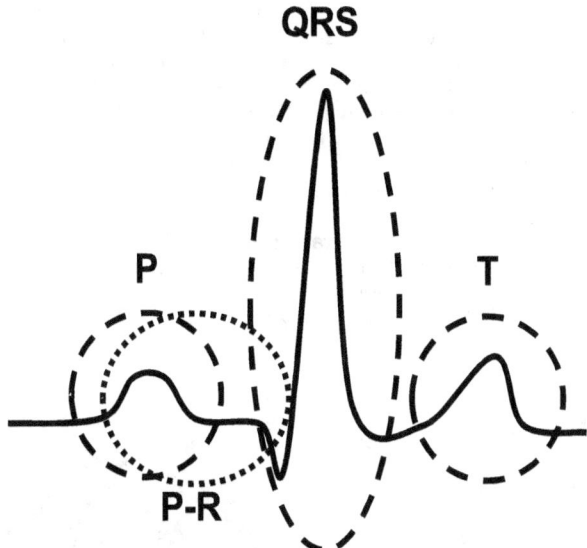

Before we begin, we should start with describing what's known as the "baseline" (or the iso-electric line as it is sometimes known as) of the ECG. This is an imaginary line drawn horizontally through the recorded ECG rhythm. All impulses should start and finish on this imaginary line. I.e. The normal P wave impulse should start on the baseline and also end on the baseline.

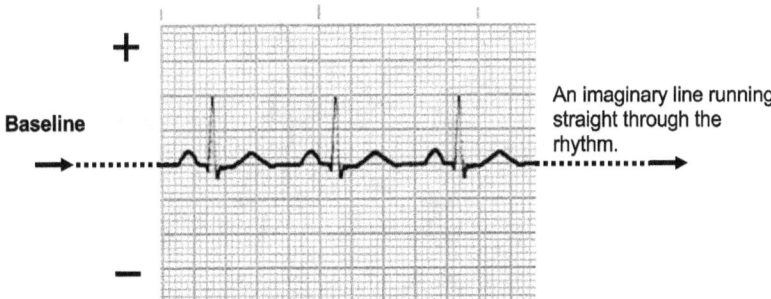

Baseline

An imaginary line running straight through the rhythm.

The Normal P Wave

The first part of any complex should be the **Normal P** wave. This shows up looking like a small hump and must be at the start of any complex, it should also be upright telling you that it is a positive signal. This is the Sino-Atrial (or SA node) node and the atriums firing off and depolarising, contracting and shortening (the Mexican wave across the sheet of muscle). All cells in the atria are capable of becoming the pacemaker, but the SA node has a higher frequency (or shouts the loudest!) so it overrides and controls all the others. The impulse passes from the right atria through the muscle separating the two, to the left atria via the specialised Bachmann Bundle pathway as this pathway can transmit up to 6 times faster than cell to cell spread. It moves from superior to inferior (top to bottom) of the atria and as the P wave tails off, the impulse now reaches the AV node. P waves are normally positive (upright) in leads I, II and V_4 to V_6. It will be negative in aVR and could either be positive or negative in any other leads.

Atrial abnormalities can be structural (right atria) or conduction (left atria) defects. These are explained in more detail on the next page. The way to tell if there is an atrial abnormality, you need a 12 lead ECG to look at leads II and V_1 for which one it is.

P wave is made up of the two chambers, which are activated separately. The right is contracted via the signal from SA node and the left is through the fast Bachman Bundle. Because of the speed of depolarisation, both signals morph into the one positive P wave.

Lead II will look directly at the natural pathway for the electrical conduction and shows as a positive P wave.

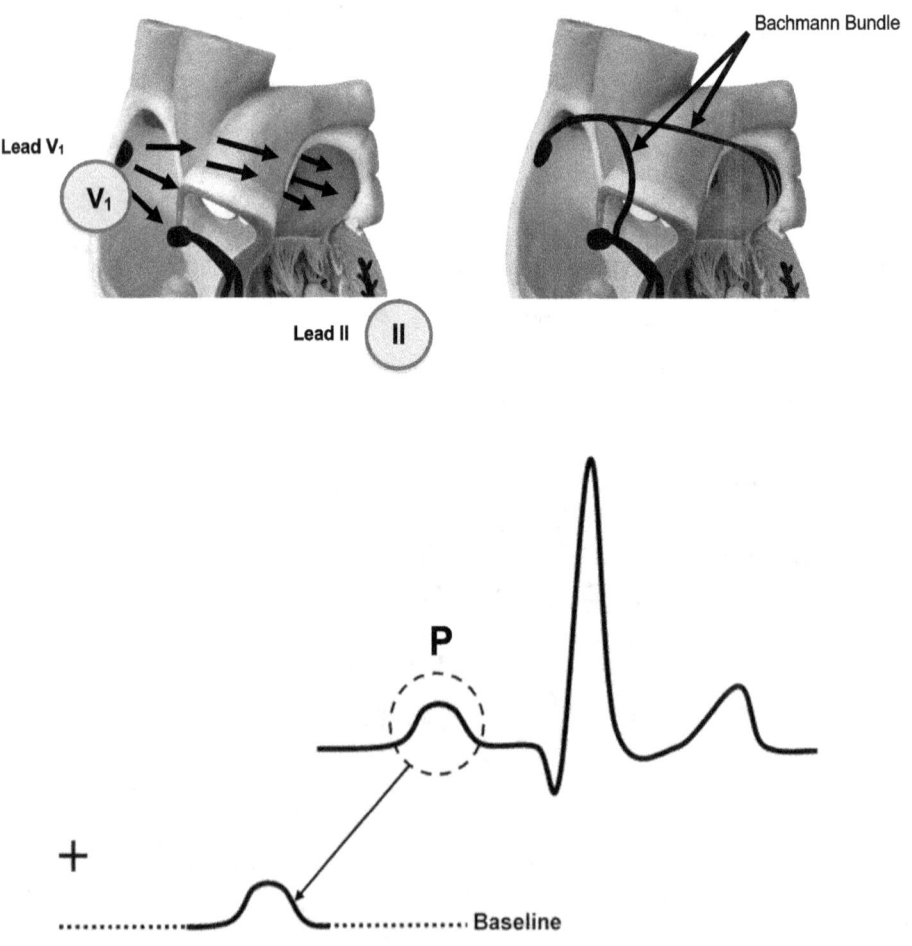

The PR interval

There is now a small delay in the conduction process in the AV node to allow the ventricles to relax and have time to fill with blood from the atria. This shows up on the ECG as the **PR** interval. It should be **no longer** than 3 to 5 small squares (0.20 secs) from the **start** of the P wave to the start of the QRS complex, which is the QRS complex. If there is an excessive delay, then there is a problem with the AV node, in which case the PR interval will be **longer** than 5 small squares (>0.20 secs). That could be due to maybe disease, damage or sometimes prescribed drugs.

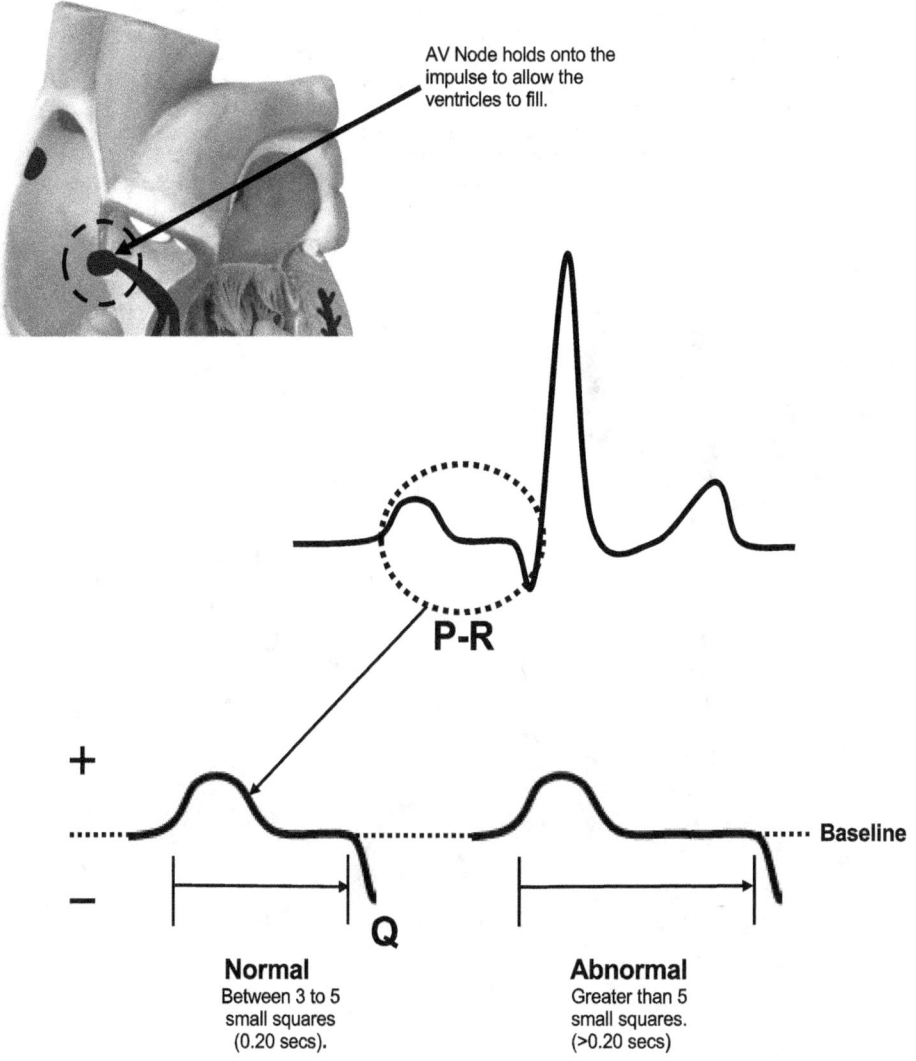

AV Node holds onto the impulse to allow the ventricles to fill.

P-R

+

−

Baseline

Q

Normal
Between 3 to 5
small squares
(0.20 secs).

Abnormal
Greater than 5
small squares.
(>0.20 secs)

The QRS Complex

The next to come along is the **QRS** complex. This is basically the straight up and down bit in the middle and the most obvious part of the ECG (this becomes very important later on) and is the impulse passing down through various parts of the ventricles. The first bit you might see is the **Q** wave, not always shown and if it is then it should be small and narrow (deep and wide Q waves usually indicate previous heart muscle death). This one is a downwards or negative deflection and is the impulse travelling from the left side bundle of HIS to the right side and septal depolarisation. Next, we see a large deflection upwards or positive and this is known as the **R** wave. This one is the impulse reaching down into the heart muscle at the bottom and up into the Purkinje fibres embedded in the heart muscle of the ventricles. The R wave then nosedives back to the baseline as the impulse reaches the Purkinje fibres, it may dip slightly below or it may not. If there is one, then this is the **S** wave, which is a downwards or negative signal. After all this, the end of the QRS complex should return to the baseline again. All of the above should be **no wider** than 3 small squares (0.12 secs) if it is a normal complex. If it is wider than this, then there is some conduction problem in the ventricles. As I mentioned above, this will become more of importance later in the book. It is at this time that the atria would also be repolarising but as the signal is so small, it is lost in the QRS complex.

As the ventricular problems are usually the most critical ones, the QRS complex can provide considerable clinical information about the condition of the heart and is, therefore, is one of the most important parts of the rhythm to be observed.

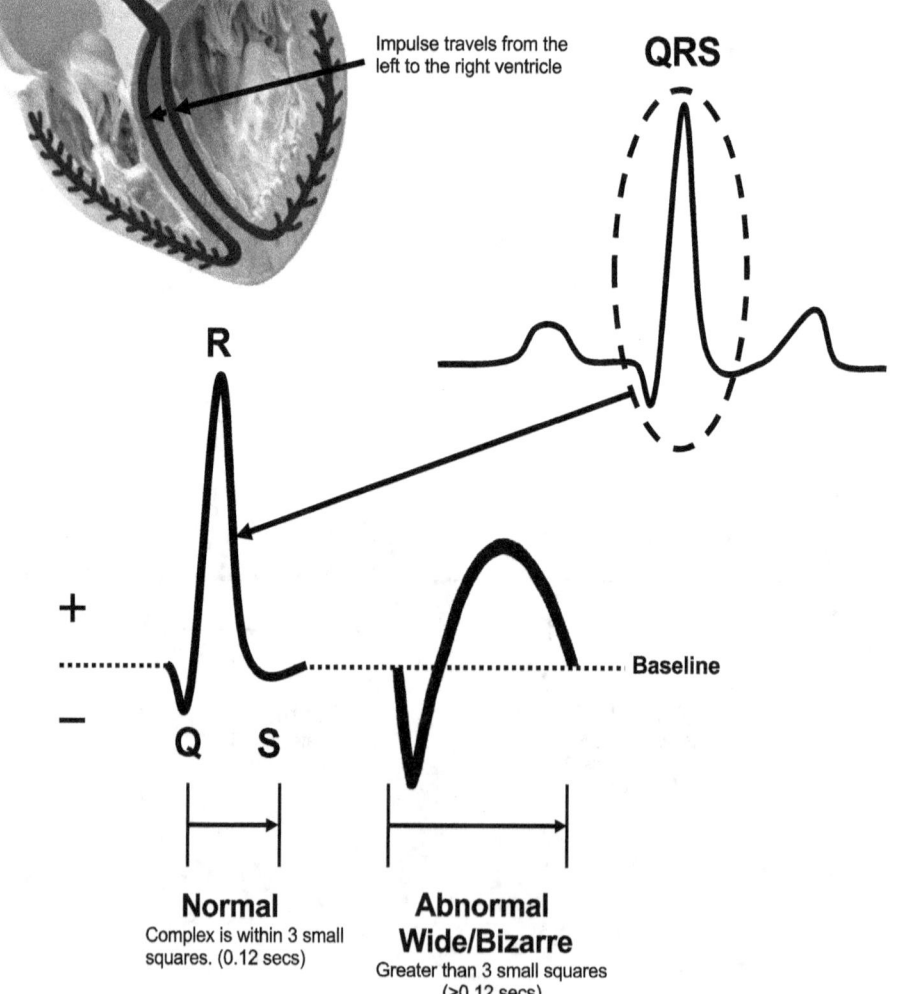

Impulse travels from the left to the right ventricle

QRS

R

+

−

Q   S

Baseline

Normal
Complex is within 3 small squares. (0.12 secs)

Abnormal
Wide/Bizarre
Greater than 3 small squares (>0.12 secs)

The T Wave

Following the QRS complex should be the **T** wave, this again should be an upward, or positive signal. It is shaped similar to the P wave but only bigger. The T wave should never be symmetrical (perfectly mirrored up stroke and down stroke) it should have a slow up stroke and a fast down stroke. This is due to the various phases that the chemicals (sodium, potassium and calcium ion channels) undergo to recharge the heart. This is the heart repolarising, or recharging ready for the next impulse (the chemical and electrical changes recharge from the inside of the heart muscle to the outside, the endocardium to the epicardium, hence the positive signal), I suppose like having a bit of a short breather before it all starts up again. This is a very sensitive and dangerous time in the ECG phase, as if you get any impulse or stimulation then it could send the heart berserk and create all sorts of problems usually resulting in a cardiac arrest. The tail end of the T wave should finish on the baseline followed by a short pause until it all starts up again!

Repolarisation

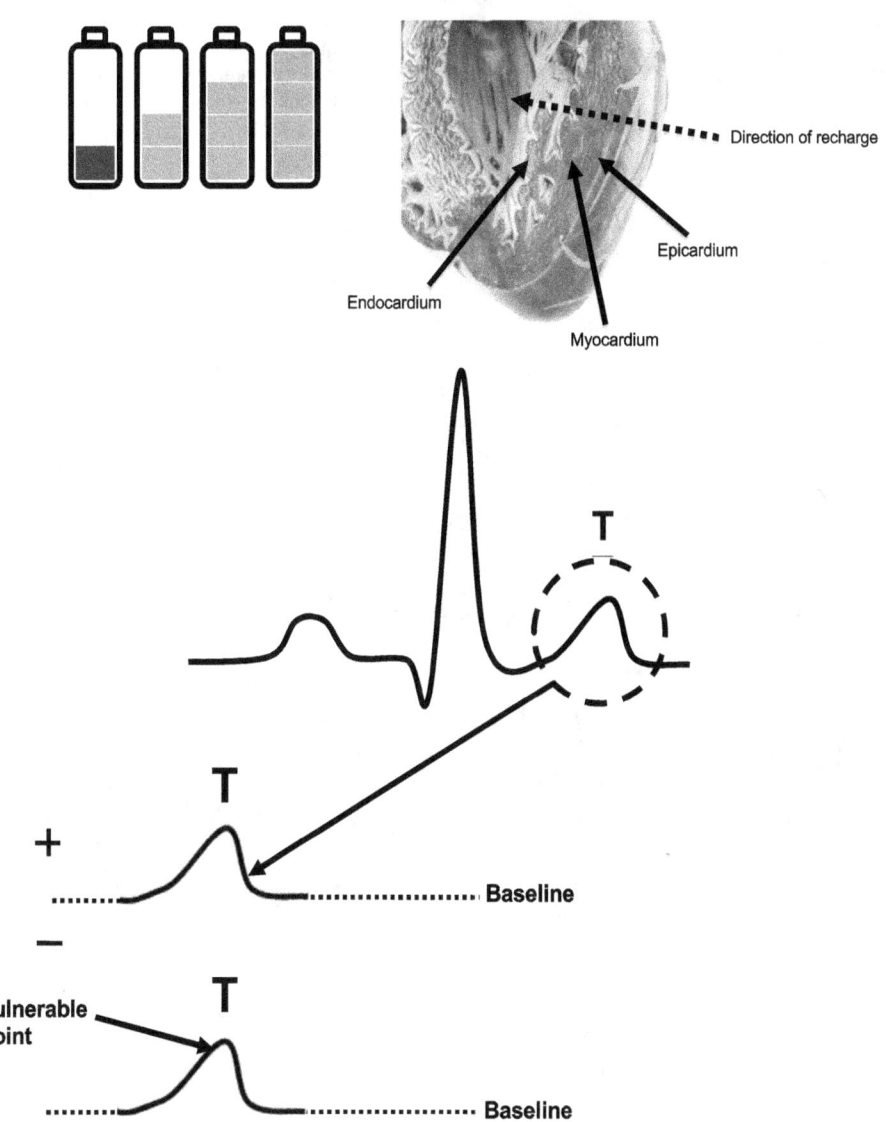

A Question of Speed

- **Question** - How on earth can you work out the rate of a rhythm?
- **Answer** - Cheat if you can and let the machine tell you, or if not then try this -

Remember, this only works out if the rhythm is regular but we can give a close guess if it is not.
The R waves are used for counting the rate, as they are the most prominent and easiest to follow.

1. Pick an R wave and count the number of **large** squares to the next one, and then divide that number by 300. For example: if there are 3 large squares between two R waves, then $300/3$ =100 BPM.
2. Another way of doing it is slight less conventional and is only a rough guide. A quick glance will tell you if the rhythm is slow or fast. Look at how many **large** squares there are between two R waves.

- In a **normal** speed rhythm (60-100 BPM), there will be between **three** and **five** large squares between R waves.
- In a **slow** rhythm (30-60), there will be between **six** and **eight** squares.
- In a **fast** rhythm (100-150 BPM), there will be between **three** and **two** squares.
- In a **very** fast rhythm (150+ BPM), there will be **one** or less large squares.

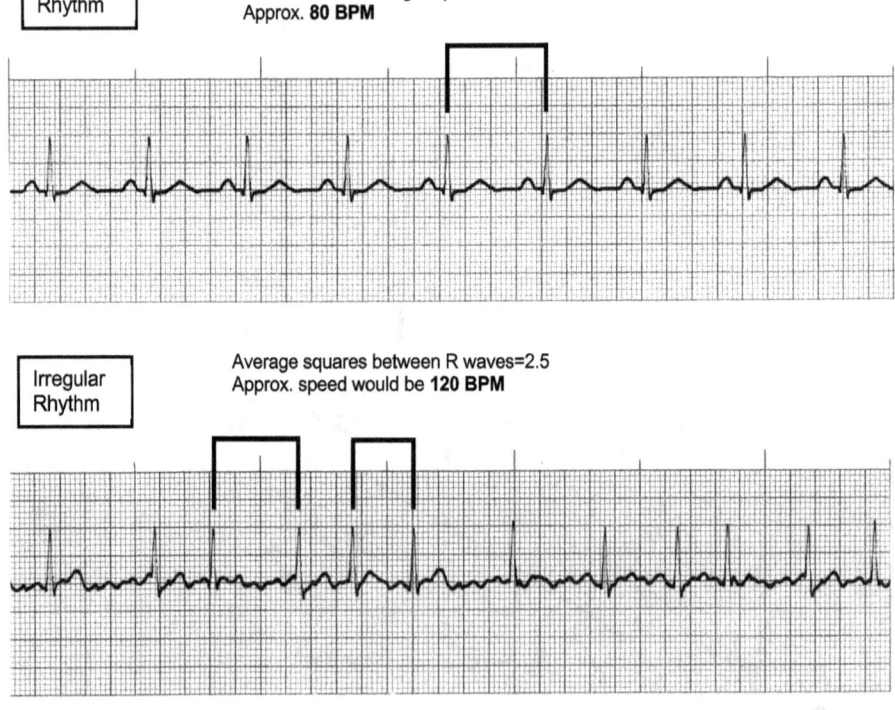

| Regular Rhythm |
Between **3** and **4** large squares between R waves =
Approx. **80 BPM**

| Irregular Rhythm |
Average squares between R waves=2.5
Approx. speed would be **120 BPM**

The simple steps to look out for on an ECG are –

- Is there a normal P wave? **Yes,** or **No**
- What Is the PR interval? Is it **Normal** (3-5 small squares gap <0.20 secs), **Long** (greater than 5 small squares gap), **Unknown** (you are not sure), or does it vary?
- Is the QRS **Normal** (<0.12 secs) or **Wide** and **Bizarre/Notched or Jagged** or does it have **Pacing spikes**?
- Is it followed by a T wave? **Yes**, **No, Abnormal** or are you **Unsure**.
- What is the rate? **Normal, Slow, Fast, V. Fast**
- What is the rhythm? Is it **Regular** or **Irregular?**

Now if you stick to these simple questions then you won't go far wrong.

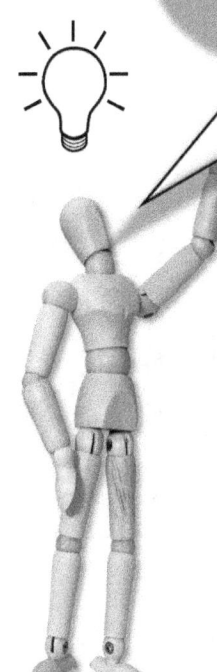

Reflect and Perfect

Ok, so we have gone through the basics of breaking down the ECG to keep it simple, but how much has actually sunk into the old grey matter?

Have a go at the questions below before you move on and you will probably be surprised at how much you actually know! The answers are upside down at the bottom of the page.

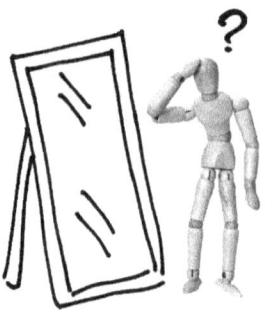

1. The P wave represents atrial depolarisation?

   True/False

2. The QRS complex represents ventricular repolarisation?

   True/False

3. The normal duration of the QRS complex should be no greater than how many secs?
   - **A.** 0.12 secs
   - **B.** 0.08 secs
   - **C.** 0.20 secs

4. The T wave represents Ventricular depolarisation?

   True/False

5. What ions make cellular electricity?
   - **A.** Sodium and Calcium with the help of Potassium
   - **B.** Sodium and Potassium with the help of Calcium
   - **C.** Calcium and Potassium with the help of sodium

6. ECG paper is printed at a speed of 50mm/sec

   True/False

7. The correct electrical conductivity pathway in the heart is:
   - **A.** P wave, AV node, Bundle of HIS, Bundle Branches, Purkinje fibres
   - **B.** P wave, Bundle of HIS, AV node, Bundle Branches, Purkinje fibres
   - **C.** P wave, Bundle Branches, Bundle of HIS, AV node, Purkinje fibres

8. The Baseline of an ECG is drawn horizontally through the ECG rhythm?

   True/False

Answers: 1. True, 2. False, 3. A, 4. False, 5. B, 6. False, 7. A, 8. True

Don't I Recognise You?

This is where we now put all of the previous learning into practice. There are 21 (yes 21!) rhythms divided into easy to digest sections (don't worry, each one is explained). At the beginning of each of these sections, you will see a comparison chart for reference. There are two more of these on page 109 which you can cut out and use if you want.

Sinus Rhythm

- Sinus Rhythm

Sinus Rhythms

- Sinus Tachycardia
- Sinus Bradycardia
- Sinus Arrhythmia

Atrial Rhythms

- Atrial Tachycardia
- Supra Ventricular Tachycardia (SVT)
- Atrial Fibrillation
- Atrial Flutter
- Atrial Ectopic

Ventricular Rhythms

- Ventricular Ectopic
- R on T Ectopic
- Bigeminal Ectopic
- Pacemaker

The Oh! Dear Rhythms

- Ventricular Tachycardia
- Ventricular Fibrillation
- Asystole

Heart Blocks

- First Degree
- Second Degree Type I (Wenckebach)
- Second Degree Type II (Mobitz)
- Third Degree
- Bundle Branch Block

Here is a comparison chart for all Atrial rhythms.

	P Waves	PR Interval	QRS	T Wave	Rate	Rhythm
Sinus Rhythm	Yes	Normal	Normal	Yes	Normal 60-100	Regular
Sinus Tachycardia	Yes	Normal	Normal	Yes	Fast 100-120	Regular
Sinus Bradycardia	Yes	Normal	Normal	Yes	Slow <60	Regular
Sinus Arrhythmia	Yes	Normal	Normal	Yes	Normal	Irregular
Atrial Tachycardia	Don't know	No	Normal	Don't know	Fast 120-140	Regular
SVT	Don't know	No	Normal	Don't know	Fast 140+	Regular
Atrial Fibrillation	F Waves	Don't know	Normal	Don't know	Fast 120+	Irregular
Atrial Flutter	Sawtoothed	Don't know	Normal	Don't know	Normal or Fast	Regular
Atrial Ectopic (Sinus)	Yes	Yes	Normal	Yes	Any	Irregular
Junctional Ectopic	No	No	Normal	Yes	Any	Irregular
First Degree Heart Block	Yes	Long	Normal	Yes	Normal	Regular
Second Degree Type One	Yes	Lengthens	Normal	Not Always	Normal	Irregular
Second Degree Type Two	Yes	Sometimes	Normal	Not Always	Normal	Regular

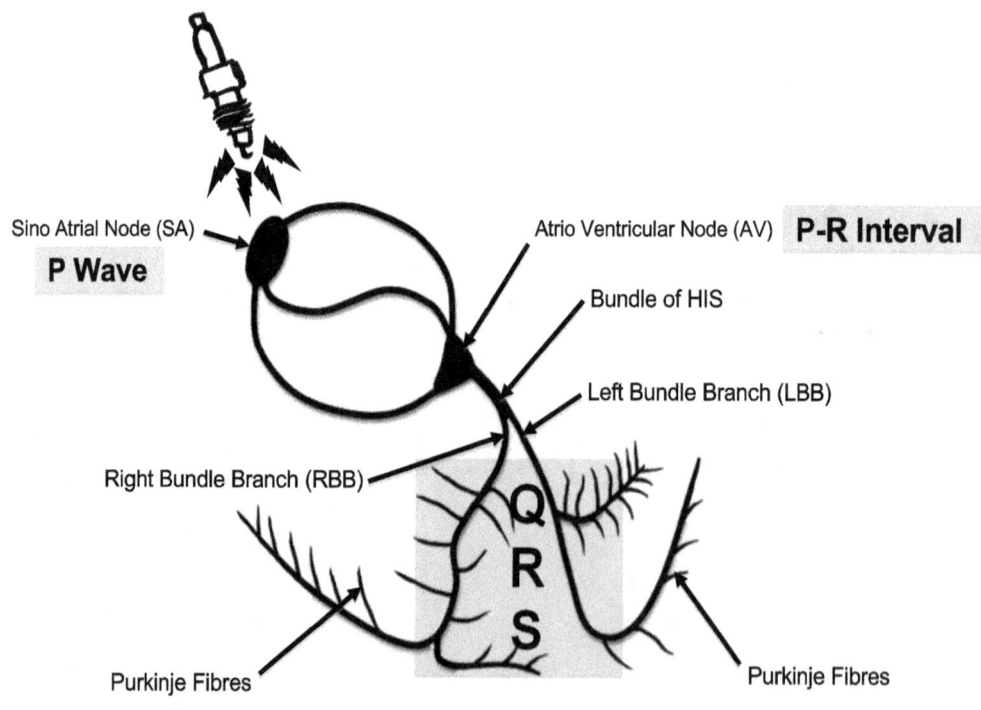

Sino Atrial Node (SA)

P Wave

Atrio Ventricular Node (AV) **P-R Interval**

Bundle of HIS

Left Bundle Branch (LBB)

Right Bundle Branch (RBB)

Q R S

Purkinje Fibres

Purkinje Fibres

Sinus Rhythm

This is where it all begins. This is the rhythm you base everything in this book on. Before we can work out what is abnormal we have to first understand what is normal. In the following rhythm, everything is normal.

	P Waves	PR Interval	QRS	T Wave	Rate	Rhythm
Sinus Rhythm	Yes	Normal	Normal	Yes	Normal 60-100	Regular
Sinus Tachycardia	Yes	Normal	Normal	Yes	Fast 100-120	Regular
Sinus Bradycardia	Yes	Normal	Normal	Yes	Slow <60	Regular
Sinus Arrhythmia	Yes	Normal	Normal	Yes	Normal	Irregular

Normal Conduction

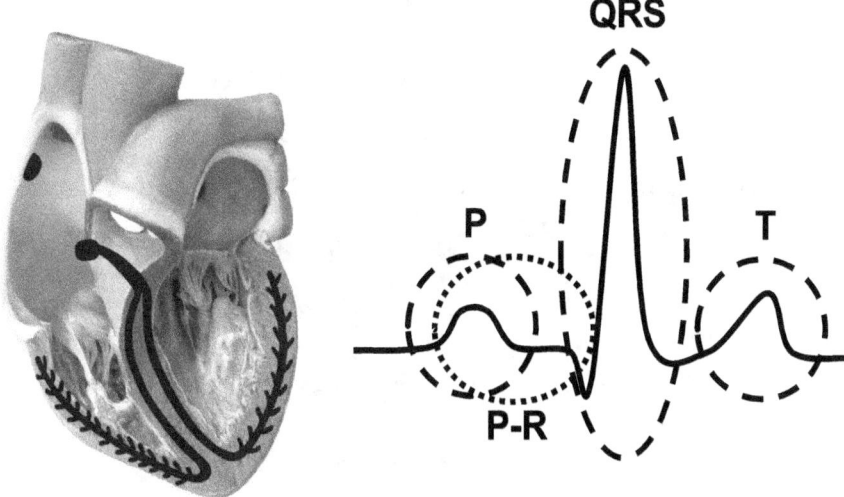

Sinus Rhythm

	P Waves	PR Interval	QRS	T Wave	Rate	Rhythm
Sinus Rhythm	Yes	Normal	Normal	Yes	Normal 60-100	Regular
Sinus Tachycardia	Yes	Normal	Normal	Yes	Fast 100-120	Regular
Sinus Bradycardia	Yes	Normal	Normal	Yes	Slow <60	Regular
Sinus Arrhythmia	Yes	Normal	Normal	Yes	Normal	Irregular

	P Waves	PR Interval	QRS	T Wave	Rate	Rhythm
Atrial Tachycardia	Don't know	No	Normal	Don't know	Fast 120-140	Regular
SVT	Don't know	No	Normal	Don't know	Fast 140+	Regular
Atrial Fibrillation	F Waves	Don't know	Normal	Don't know	Fast 120+	Irregular
Atrial Flutter	Sawtoothed	Don't know	Normal	Don't know	Normal or Fast	Regular
Atrial Ectopic (Sinus)	Yes	Yes	Normal	Yes	Normal	Irregular

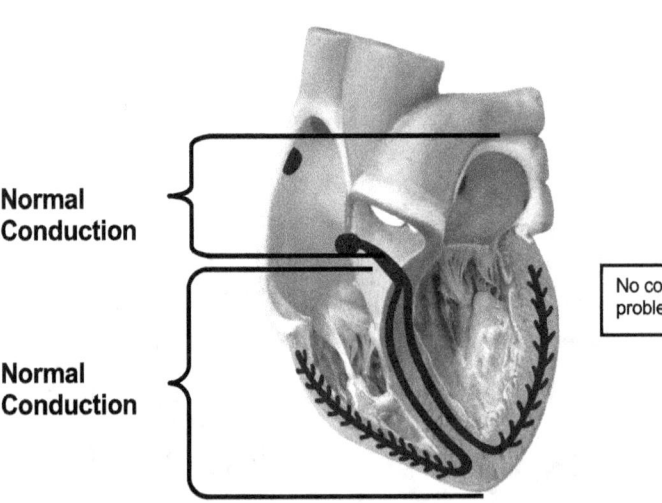

Normal Conduction

Normal Conduction

No conduction problems here

Sinus Rhythm

Here is where it all begins. The first one (and the most boring but important one) we should look at before we can do anything else. If you can work out this one, then the rest should be plain sailing (or plain driving if you don't have a boat!). The **P waves** are **normal** and they are within the correct distance from the QRS (the normal PR interval is between 3 to 5 small squares). The **QRS** complexes are also **normal**, not wide or bizarre; all this is followed by a **T wave**. Let's now have a look at the rate and the rhythm. We see that it is normal (between 60-100 BPM) and the rhythm is regular. So basically, this is now Normal Sinus Rhythm (SR as it is commonly known as). Easy isn't it? A common phrase you may have heard of is, "if it looks like a duck and quacks like a duck, then (until proven otherwise), it is a duck" So if it looks like a normal sinus rhythm then it is.

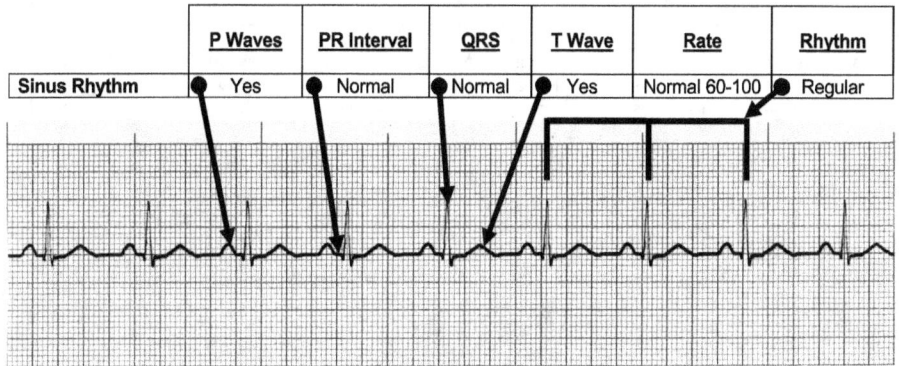

	P Waves	PR Interval	QRS	T Wave	Rate	Rhythm
Sinus Rhythm	Yes	Normal	Normal	Yes	Normal 60-100	Regular

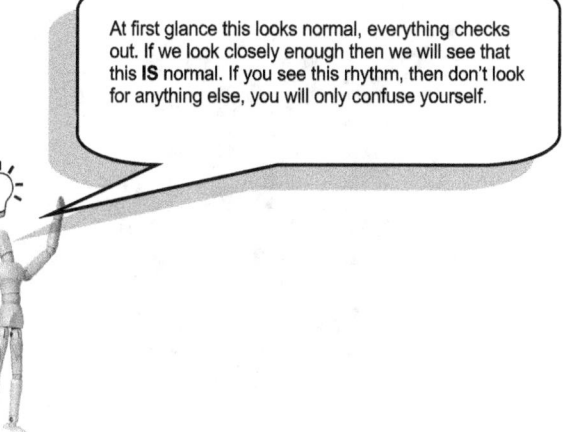

At first glance this looks normal, everything checks out. If we look closely enough then we will see that this **IS** normal. If you see this rhythm, then don't look for anything else, you will only confuse yourself.

Sinus Arrhythmias

Simply put this is a posh description of any rhythm that is an abnormal Sinus pattern. All of these rhythms originate from the Sino Atrial (SA) node so you should see the P wave. The QRS complexes are always normal.

	P Waves	PR Interval	QRS	T Wave	Rate	Rhythm
Sinus Rhythm	Yes	Normal	Normal	Yes	Normal 60-100	Regular
Sinus Tachycardia	Yes	Normal	Normal	Yes	Fast 100-120	Regular
Sinus Bradycardia	Yes	Normal	Normal	Yes	Slow <60	Regular
Sinus Arrhythmia	Yes	Normal	Normal	Yes	Normal	Irregular

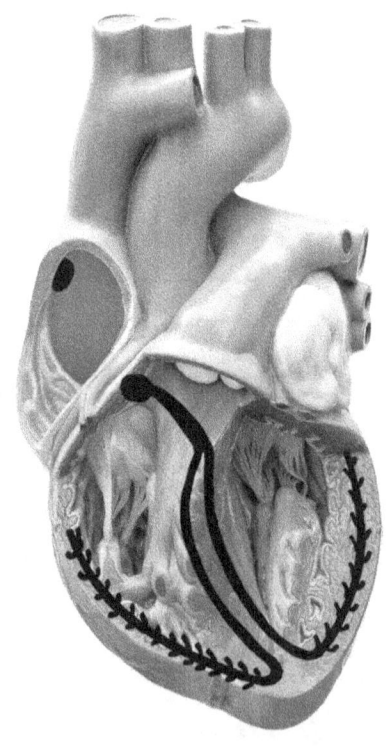

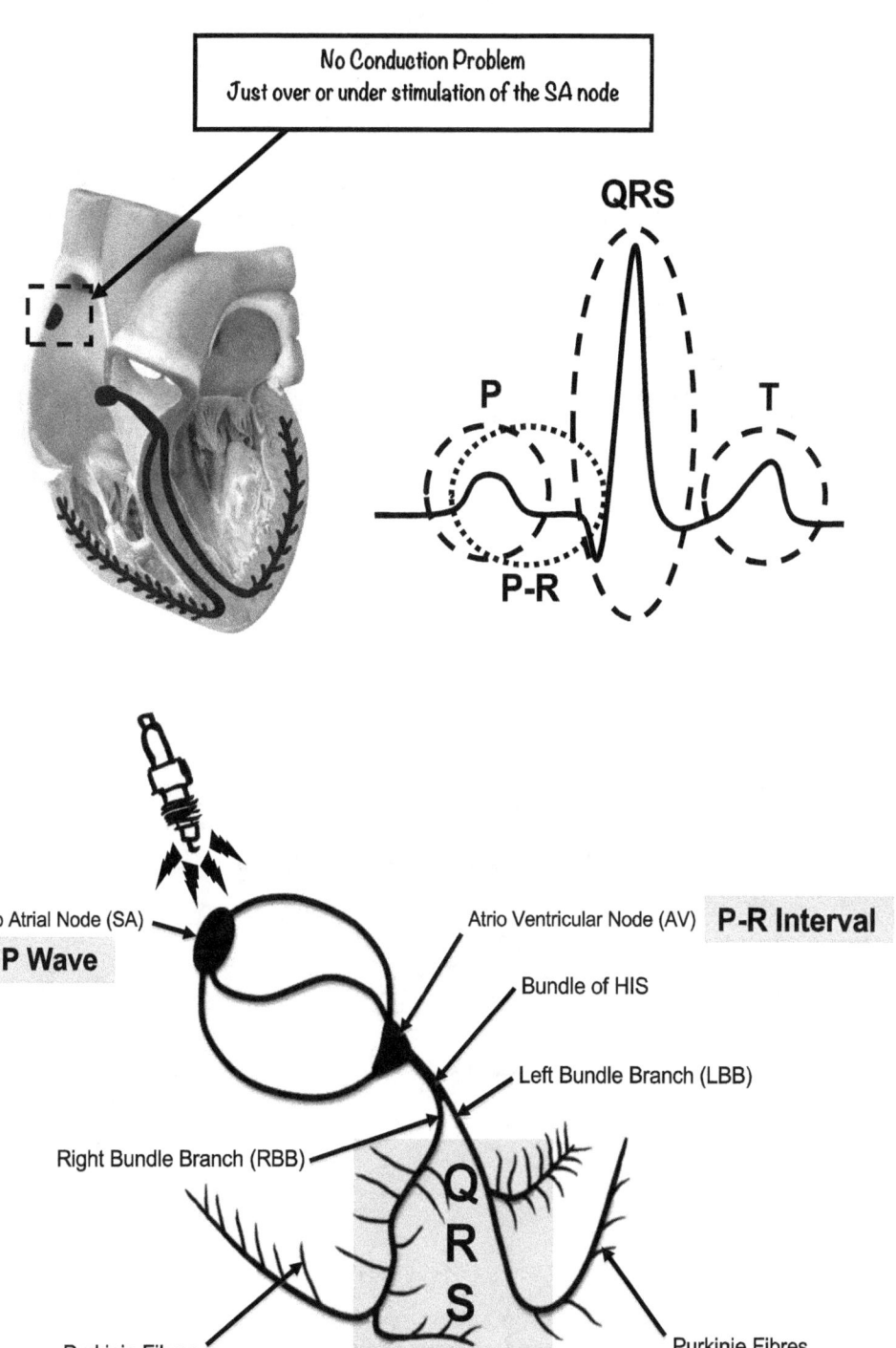

Sinus Tachycardia

	P Waves	PR Interval	QRS	T Wave	Rate	Rhythm
Sinus Rhythm	Yes	Normal	Normal	Yes	Normal 60-100	Regular
Sinus Tachycardia	Yes	Normal	Normal	Yes	Fast 100-120	Regular
Sinus Bradycardia	Yes	Normal	Normal	Yes	Slow <60	Regular
Sinus Arrhythmia	Yes	Normal	Normal	Yes	Normal	Irregular
Atrial Tachycardia	Don't know	No	Normal	Don't know	Fast 120-140	Regular
SVT	Don't know	No	Normal	Don't know	Fast 140+	Regular
Atrial Fibrillation	F Waves	Don't know	Normal	Don't know	Fast 120+	Irregular
Atrial Flutter	Sawtoothed	Don't know	Normal	Don't know	Normal or Fast	Regular
Atrial Ectopic (Sinus)	Yes	Yes	Normal	Yes	Any	Irregular
Junctional Ectopic	No	No	Normal	Yes	Any	Irregular

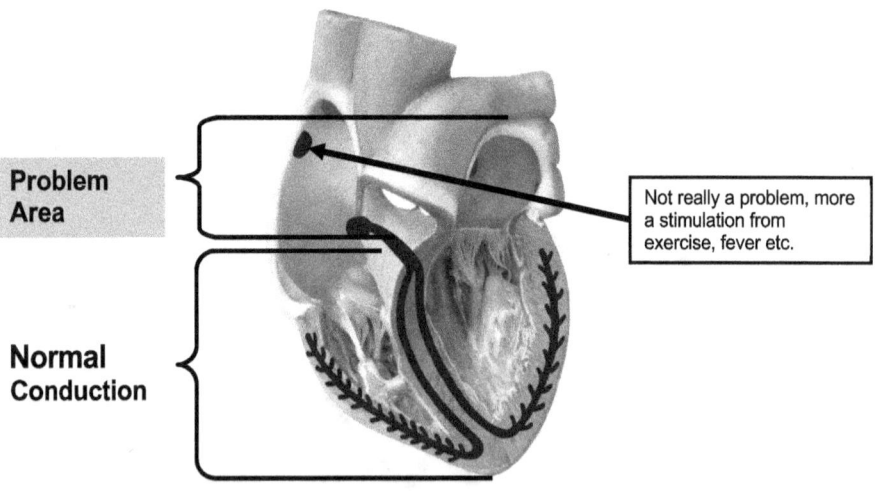

Problem Area

Normal Conduction

Not really a problem, more a stimulation from exercise, fever etc.

Sinus Tachycardia (ST)

Basically, the underlying rhythm is sinus rhythm. There is a normal P wave, the PR interval is normal this is followed by a normal QRS, then a T wave, but it is just a bit faster than 100 BPM which is classed as an inappropriately rapid rate. There will be two basic types of sinus tachycardia, the ones where it gradually accelerates to a rapid rate and then deaccelerates when the problem has been removed or treated. Some of these will be the ones that would be pain, fever, shock, cocaine or other stimulant drugs, heart failure or exercise (running down to the pub before last orders!) and other would be the instantaneous cause such as an unexpected loud noise, anxiety, or anything that would cause a sudden and rapid increase in heart rate. You will find that after resting or treatment, this rhythm should usually return to normal after the underlying problem has been resolved. If not, then you need to look for the root medical or physical cause of the problem.

	P Waves	PR Interval	QRS	T Wave	Rate	Rhythm
Sinus Tachycardia	Yes	Normal	Normal	Yes	Fast 100-120	Regular

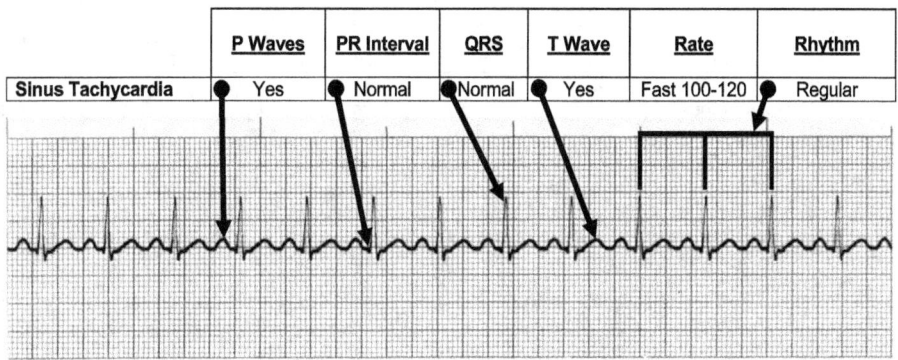

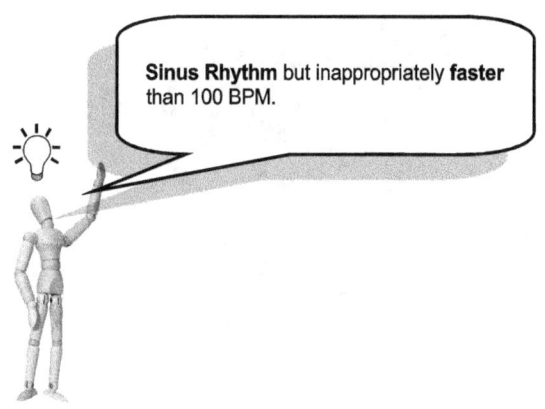

Sinus Rhythm but inappropriately **faster** than 100 BPM.

Sinus Bradycardia

	P Waves	PR Interval	QRS	T Wave	Rate	Rhythm
Sinus Rhythm	Yes	Normal	Normal	Yes	Normal 60-100	Regular
Sinus Tachycardia	Yes	Normal	Normal	Yes	Fast 100-120	Regular
Sinus Bradycardia	Yes	Normal	Normal	Yes	Slow <60	Regular
Sinus Arrhythmia	Yes	Normal	Normal	Yes	Normal	Irregular

	P Waves	PR Interval	QRS	T Wave	Rate	Rhythm
Atrial Tachycardia	Don't know	No	Normal	Don't know	Fast 120-140	Regular
SVT	Don't know	No	Normal	Don't know	Fast 140+	Regular
Atrial Fibrillation	F Waves	Don't know	Normal	Don't know	Fast 120+	Irregular
Atrial Flutter	Sawtoothed	Don't know	Normal	Don't know	Normal or Fast	Regular
Atrial Ectopic (Sinus)	Yes	Yes	Normal	Yes	Any	Irregular
Junctional Ectopic	No	No	Normal	Yes	Any	Irregular

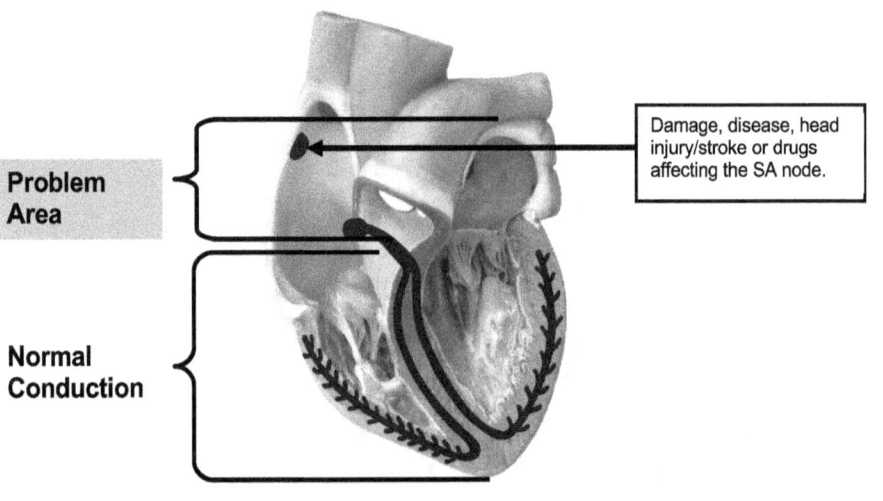

Problem Area

Normal Conduction

Damage, disease, head injury/stroke or drugs affecting the SA node.

Sinus Bradycardia

This one is more obvious than most. Sinus Rhythm apart from the fact that it is a lot slower, less than 60 BPM (Some define this differently but most will class true Bradycardia as less than 50 BPM). This may be normal in a fit and athletic person (well not me for a start, that sound like too much hard work!), with some athletes having a normal pulse rate in the 40's or even lower. Other causes may be due to a faint (Syncope), disease or damage to the SA node due to age and blood supply problems, hypothermia, head injury or haemorrhage. It could also be caused by some prescribed drugs and can commonly occur during sleep. Also, if you vomit, or if you have constipation or strain to open your bowels can cause bradycardia or worse as you cause a Valsalva (named after a17th century physician and anatomist called Antonio Maria Valsalva) manoeuvre. This will increase the abdominal pressure which helps to force out the stools. As a consequence of this, whilst bearing down you hold your breath which causes an increase in your chest which reduces the blood flow to your heart. That is why many people with cardiac problems die on the toilet!

In most cases the heart rhythm should return to normal again as soon as the problem is resolved. Worth mentioning too is that this is one of the common rhythms you may see after an MI (myocardial infarction or heart attack) or stroke (CVA - Cerebral Vascular Attack).

Unless it is symptomatic (red flag or concerning symptoms) then Sinus Bradycardia is not usually treated when drugs or a pacemaker may be considered.

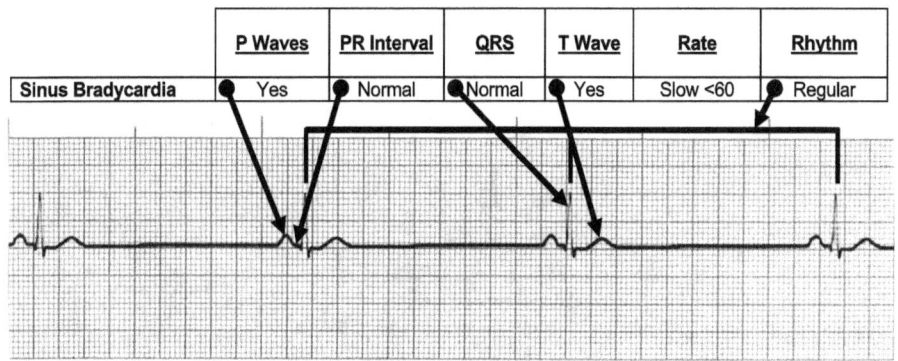

	P Waves	PR Interval	QRS	T Wave	Rate	Rhythm
Sinus Bradycardia	Yes	Normal	Normal	Yes	Slow <60	Regular

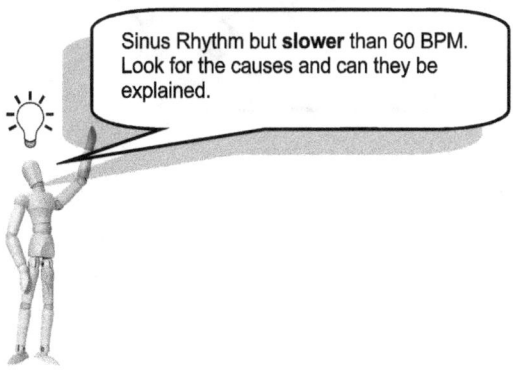

Sinus Rhythm but **slower** than 60 BPM. Look for the causes and can they be explained.

Sinus Arrhythmia

	P Waves	PR Interval	QRS	T Wave	Rate	Rhythm
Sinus Rhythm	Yes	Normal	Normal	Yes	Normal 60-100	Regular
Sinus Tachycardia	Yes	Normal	Normal	Yes	Fast 100-120	Regular
Sinus Bradycardia	Yes	Normal	Normal	Yes	Slow <60	Regular
Sinus Arrhythmia	Yes	Normal	Normal	Yes	Normal	Irregular
Atrial Tachycardia	Don't know	No	Normal	Don't know	Fast 120-140	Regular
SVT	Don't know	No	Normal	Don't know	Fast 140+	Regular
Atrial Fibrillation	F Waves	Don't know	Normal	Don't know	Fast 120+	Irregular
Atrial Flutter	Sawtoothed	Don't know	Normal	Don't know	Normal or Fast	Regular
Atrial Ectopic (Sinus)	Yes	Yes	Normal	Yes	Any	Irregular
Junctional Ectopic	No	No	Normal	Yes	Any	Irregular

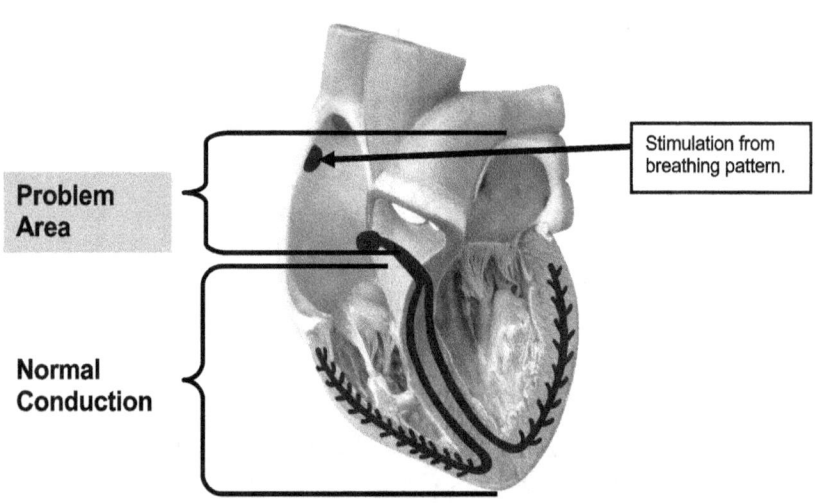

Stimulation from breathing pattern.

Problem Area

Normal Conduction

Sinus Arrhythmia

Sinus rhythm apart for small periods when the heart rate suddenly increases for a brief time then goes back to normal. The SA node gets stimulated a bit more as you breathe in and relaxes down when you breathe out. This is perfectly normal and is due to the increased intrathoracic pressure in the chest cavity. It is especially noticeable in children, athletes and young adults and nothing to worry about. Have a go on yourself or someone suitable that you know (please warn them first that it does not mean that they may have a cardiac condition!), take your pulse and breathe in and out slowly and deeply then see if you pulse changes. It should slow down when you breathe out and speed up when you breathe in.

Anyway, look at your patient, when they breathe in does the heart rate increase and when they breathe out does it return to normal? If it does, then there is your answer.

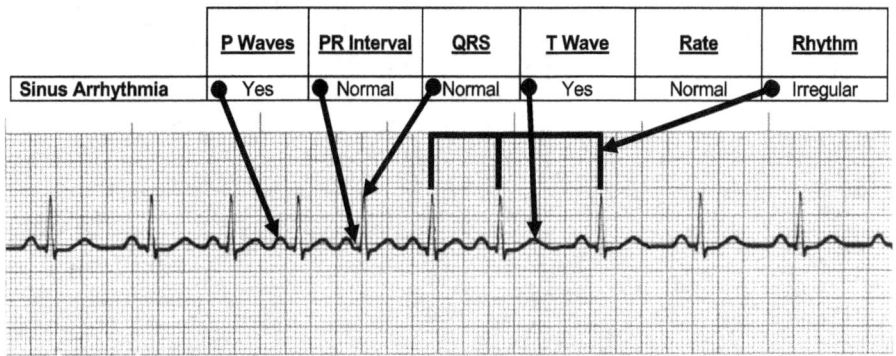

	P Waves	PR Interval	QRS	T Wave	Rate	Rhythm
Sinus Arrhythmia	Yes	Normal	Normal	Yes	Normal	Irregular

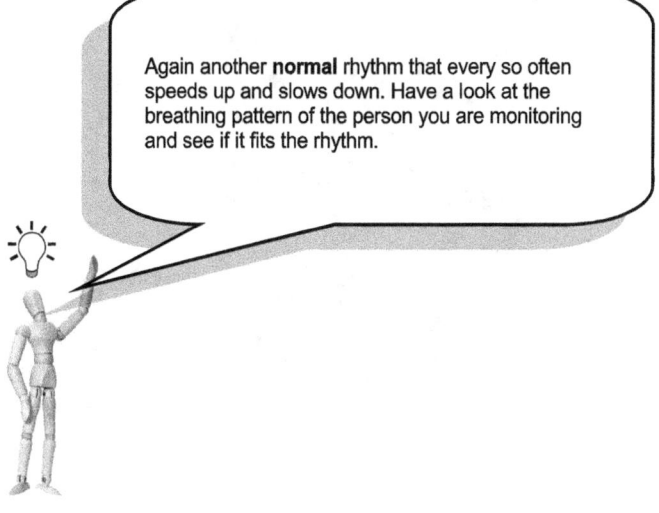

Again another **normal** rhythm that every so often speeds up and slows down. Have a look at the breathing pattern of the person you are monitoring and see if it fits the rhythm.

Atrial Arrhythmias

Looking at these ones, you will find that the QRS is normal and it is the P wave, which is playing up.

	P Waves	PR Interval	QRS	T Wave	Rate	Rhythm
Atrial Tachycardia	Don't know	No	Normal	Don't know	Fast 120-140	Regular
SVT	Don't know	No	Normal	Don't know	Fast 140+	Regular
Atrial Fibrillation	F Waves	Don't know	Normal	Don't know	Fast 120+	Irregular
Atrial Flutter	Sawtoothed	Don't know	Normal	Don't know	Normal or Fast	Regular
Atrial Ectopic (Sinus)	Yes	Yes	Normal	Yes	Normal	Irregular
Junctional Ectopic	No	No	Normal	Yes	Normal	Irregular

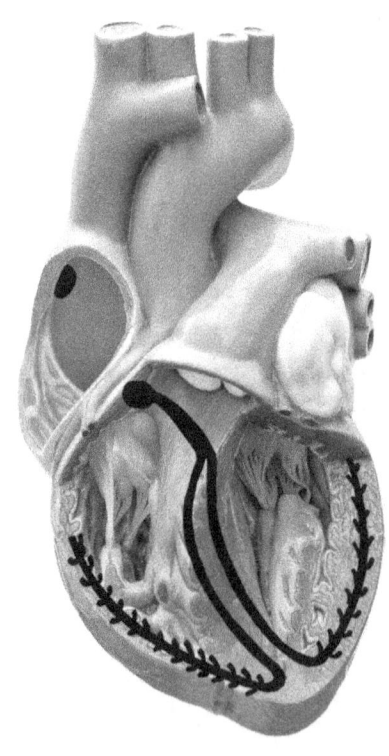

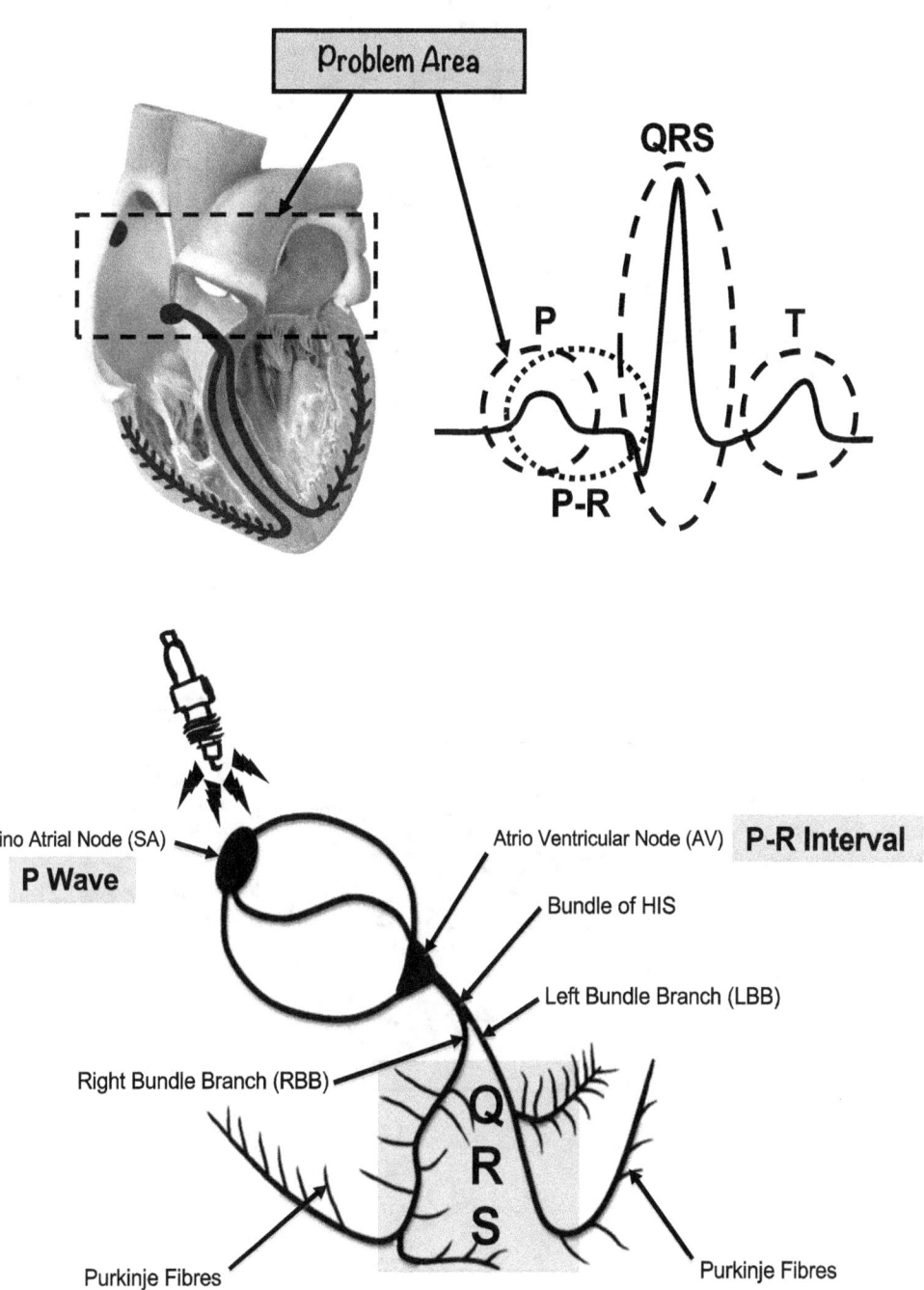

Problem Area

QRS

P

P-R

T

Sino Atrial Node (SA)

P Wave

Atrio Ventricular Node (AV)

P-R Interval

Bundle of HIS

Left Bundle Branch (LBB)

Right Bundle Branch (RBB)

Q
R
S

Purkinje Fibres

Purkinje Fibres

Atrial Tachycardia

	P Waves	PR Interval	QRS	T Wave	Rate	Rhythm
Sinus Rhythm	Yes	Normal	Normal	Yes	Normal 60-100	Regular
Sinus Tachycardia	Yes	Normal	Normal	Yes	Fast 100-120	Regular
Sinus Bradycardia	Yes	Normal	Normal	Yes	Slow <60	Regular
Sinus Arrhythmia	Yes	Normal	Normal	Yes	Normal	Irregular

	P Waves	PR Interval	QRS	T Wave	Rate	Rhythm
Atrial Tachycardia	Don't know	No	Normal	Don't know	Fast 120-140	Regular
SVT	Don't know	No	Normal	Don't know	Fast 140+	Regular
Atrial Fibrillation	F Waves	Don't know	Normal	Don't know	Fast 120+	Irregular
Atrial Flutter	Sawtoothed	Don't know	Normal	Don't know	Normal or Fast	Regular
Atrial Ectopic (Sinus)	Yes	Yes	Normal	Yes	Normal	Irregular
Junctional Ectopic	No	No	Normal	Yes	Normal	Irregular

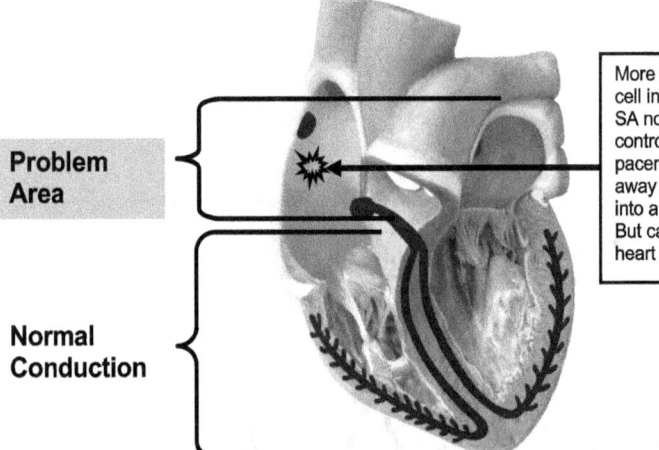

Problem Area

More commonly a focal cell in the Atria near the SA node that has taken control as the pacemaker and has run away a bit fast and gone into a re-entry pattern. But can be caused by heart defects or drugs.

Normal Conduction

Atrial Tachycardia

This is a fast regular rhythm usually running >120 BPM. The most obvious thing with this rhythm is the speed and regularity. The difficulty is the bit in-between the QRS complexes, they appear to be abnormally shaped P waves (or are they T waves?). The fast ventricular rate makes it difficult to work out where the impulse is coming from. The SA node is overpowered by a possible re-entry focus that is normally located in the pulmonary veins or the crista terminalis (a vertical ridge of smooth myocardial muscle located within the right atrium of the heart). The P wave is buried in the T wave (because of the speed) giving it that notchy appearance. Again, the root cause can sometimes explain many reasons for this rhythm. This could be the heart compensating for blood loss in stage four shock; it could be accelerants such as cocaine, stimulant caffeine and energy drinks, amphetamines or other prescription or non-prescription drugs. This also could be a structure heart problem such atrial disease/dilation or mitral valve stenosis.

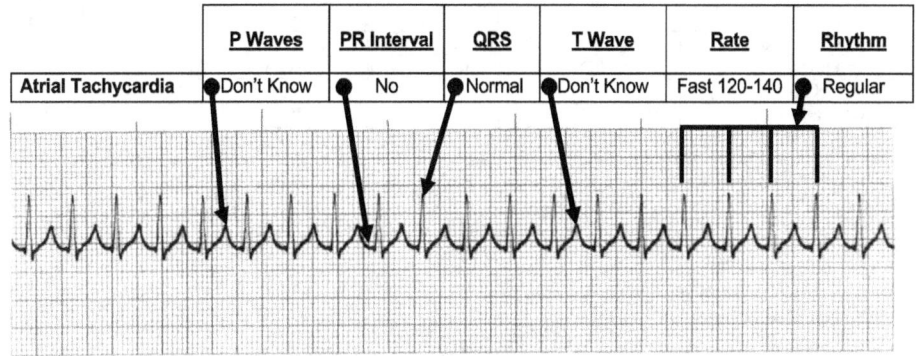

	P Waves	PR Interval	QRS	T Wave	Rate	Rhythm
Atrial Tachycardia	Don't Know	No	Normal	Don't Know	Fast 120-140	Regular

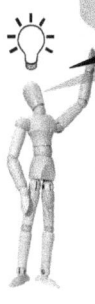

A fast, regular atrial rhythm >100 BPM from a focus outside the SA node or a possible re-entry circuit. There are no obvious P or T waves, they seem to be buried in each other.

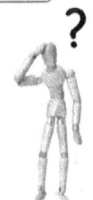

Supra Ventricular Tachycardia

	P Waves	PR Interval	QRS	T Wave	Rate	Rhythm
Sinus Rhythm	Yes	Normal	Normal	Yes	Normal 60-100	Regular
Sinus Tachycardia	Yes	Normal	Normal	Yes	Fast 100-120	Regular
Sinus Bradycardia	Yes	Normal	Normal	Yes	Slow <60	Regular
Sinus Arrhythmia	Yes	Normal	Normal	Yes	Normal	Irregular

	P Waves	PR Interval	QRS	T Wave	Rate	Rhythm
Atrial Tachycardia	Don't know	No	Normal	Don't know	Fast 120-140	Regular
SVT	Don't know	No	Normal	Don't know	Fast 140+	Regular
Atrial Fibrillation	F Waves	Don't know	Normal	Don't know	Fast 120+	Irregular
Atrial Flutter	Sawtoothed	Don't know	Normal	Don't know	Normal or Fast	Regular
Atrial Ectopic (Sinus)	Yes	Yes	Normal	Yes	Normal	Irregular
Junctional Ectopic	No	No	Normal	Yes	Normal	Irregular

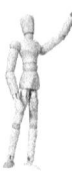

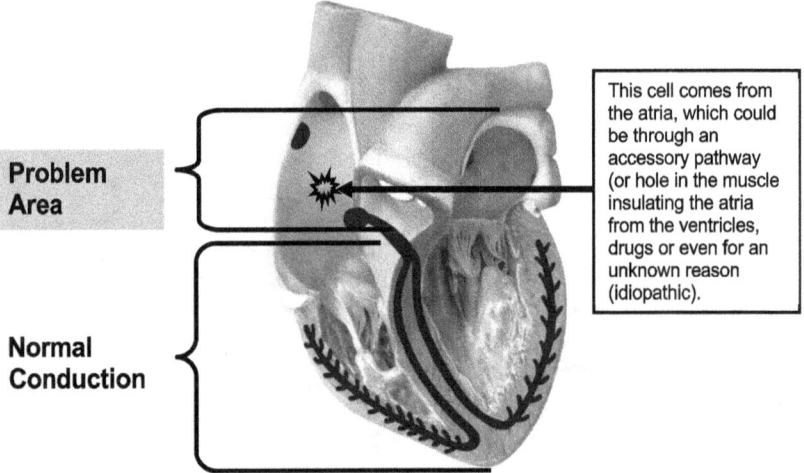

Problem Area

Normal Conduction

This cell comes from the atria, which could be through an accessory pathway (or hole in the muscle insulating the atria from the ventricles, drugs or even for an unknown reason (idiopathic).

Supra Ventricular Tachycardia (SVT)

S.V.T, short for Supra-Ventricular-Tachycardia. It sounds more like a Japanese sports car doesn't it? Actually, it's a complicated name for something quite simple. Supra means above, so Supra Ventricular means above the ventricles. Tachycardia, as you know, means it is a fast rhythm (greater than 100 BPM). So SVT is a fast rhythm originating from above the ventricles, simple isn't it?

This one could be due to a number of problems, which could be drugs overdose (especially cocaine or stimulants again), SA or AV node damage, a re-entry, or it could just simply happen for no reason whatsoever (this is called idiopathic). It is also a possibility that it could be from an accessory pathway (a hole in the insulating muscle between the atria and the ventricles) and does not go down the correctly determined pathway; this will start to depolarise the ventricles too early (called pre-excitement) due to the "leak" in the insulation. Causes of this could be a genetic condition such as Wolfe Parkinson White Syndrome (WPW).

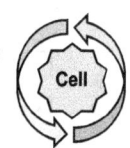

Unfortunately, this is not one of your easiest rhythms to work out. As with the tachys, Sinus tachy is usually >100 to 120 BPM, Atrial tachy is about >120 to 160 and SVT runs at about >140 to 180 so with the overlap it makes it harder to determine so this rhythm can be a bit difficult to work out as sometimes it's not easy to tell whether it is Atrial Tachy or Ventricular Tachycardia or VT (see pages 47 + 73). The impulse could get a bundle branch block in the ventricles and could widen the QRS complex **and** make them wide and bizarre at the higher speeds. VT is classed as a slightly irregular rhythm, while SVT is regular. If in doubt go for the worst, then you will not have an unpleasant surprise.

	P Waves	PR Interval	QRS	T Wave	Rate	Rhythm
SVT	●Don't know	● No	●Normal	●Don't know	Fast 140+	● Regular

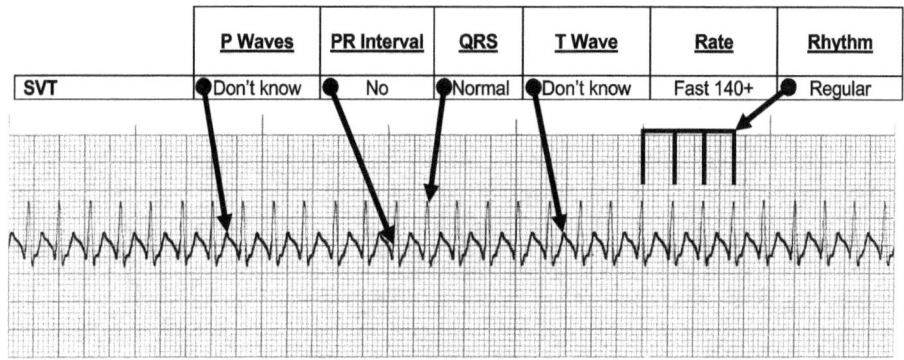

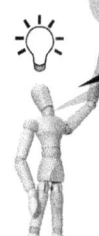

This is a very fast rhythm, usually regular. It can become difficult to tell SVT from Ventricular Tachycardia (VT) as the ventricular impulse could get distorted at the fastest speeds and the QRS complexes become wide and bizarre. If you can't tell, then treat it as VT.

Atrial Fibrillation

	P Waves	PR Interval	QRS	T Wave	Rate	Rhythm
Sinus Rhythm	Yes	Normal	Normal	Yes	Normal 60-100	Regular
Sinus Tachycardia	Yes	Normal	Normal	Yes	Fast 100-120	Regular
Sinus Bradycardia	Yes	Normal	Normal	Yes	Slow <60	Regular
Sinus Arrhythmia	Yes	Normal	Normal	Yes	Normal	Irregular
Atrial Tachycardia	Don't know	No	Normal	Don't know	Fast 120-140	Regular
SVT	Don't know	No	Normal	Don't know	Fast 140+	Regular
Atrial Fibrillation	F Waves	Don't know	Normal	Don't know	Fast 120+	Irregular
Atrial Flutter	Sawtoothed	Don't know	Normal	Don't know	Normal or Fast	Regular
Atrial Ectopic (Sinus)	Yes	Yes	Normal	Yes	Normal	Irregular
Junctional Ectopic	No	No	Normal	Yes	Normal	Irregular

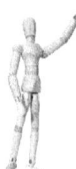

Problem Area

Normal Conduction

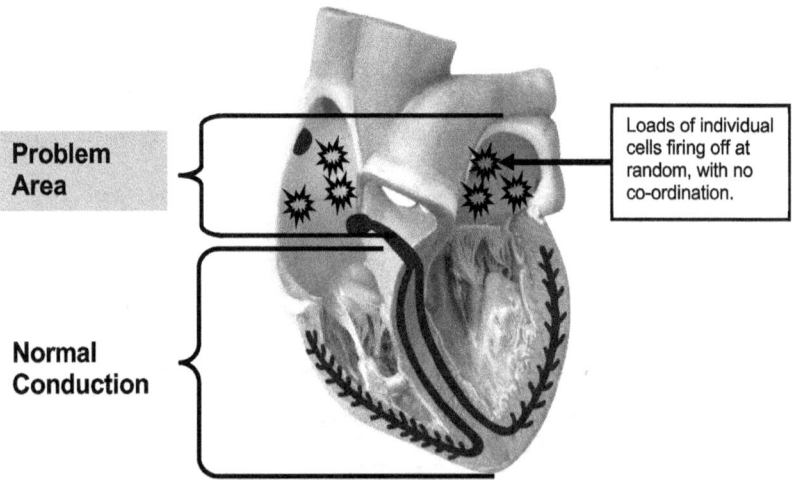

Loads of individual cells firing off at random, with no co-ordination.

Atrial Fibrillation (AF)

Usually a fast rhythm and can be fairly easy to recognise due to its **speed** and **irregularity** (especially the P waves). It tends to be one of the most common abnormal rhythms that you are likely to come across. The first thing to do is to rule out any muscle tremor or interference beforehand. This rhythm is commonly caused by hypertension, diabetes, valvular heart disease and Congenital Heart Disease. Fibrosis of the atria from dilation or genetics can enhance the chances of atrial fibrillation.

It seems that to the atria, the SA node has been disabled and the cells (usually dominated by the left atrium and around the aortic and pulmonary valve area) in the atrial wall are having their own private re-entry party. This causes mass hysteria in the atria and because there is no Mexican Wave (page 14) and no normal P wave, the atria sit there and quiver to themselves and don't pump. This shows up on the ECG as uncoordinated and undiscernible P wave, it is difficult to tell if they are P or T waves, so they are called Fibrillation or Flutter (F) waves (not my idea!).

The impulses (or wavelets) and are usually as high as 600 per minute but many of these reach the AV node. The AV node in the meantime is working normally bit is getting confused as it is not getting its usual supply of steady impulses, so what it does is it grabs the strongest wavelets that come along and conducts these through the normal conductive pathway, making the QRS complexes very irregular in rhythm but narrow < 0.12 msec or < 3 small squares which conducts through to the ventricles. This is a common rhythm for someone who has had a recent stroke and more common in the elderly as 95% of the SA node function is lost over the age of 75. Intense, prolonged physical training in sports such as triathlon or iron man competitions have been known to be a contributing factor to the early onset of AF as the SA node is bombarded with sustained activity due to the intensity of the training and exercise. 21% of AF sufferers are asymptomatic and most people who suffer from it suffer bouts, then normality (paroxysmal AF), so some people may not even know that they have this heart condition. It is important thing to remember that due to the loss of the atrial pumping action, then anyone who suffers from AF then will have difficulty sleeping lying down because when the heart is placed horizontally (lying on their back usually with no or not many pillows) and with no atrial pumping, then the ventricles will find it harder to fill making it work harder, faster and less effective causing possible shortness of breath and discomfort. So the best advice is for someone to sleep sitting more upright allowing gravity to fill the ventricles and reduce the workload on the heart. This problem can sometimes be cardioverted if the first onset is within 24 hours, or maybe even resolved by ablating (or using surgical alcohol to "burn" away the irritation). This is not always successful as the AF can return and also it can cause further complications. Statistically, women with AF have a worse prognosis than men. Also interestingly enough, you can get this condition from binge alcohol drinking. This is known as "holiday heart syndrome"!

	P Waves	PR Interval	QRS	T Wave	Rate	Rhythm
Atrial Fibrillation	F Waves	Don't know	Normal	Don't know	Fast 120+	Irregular

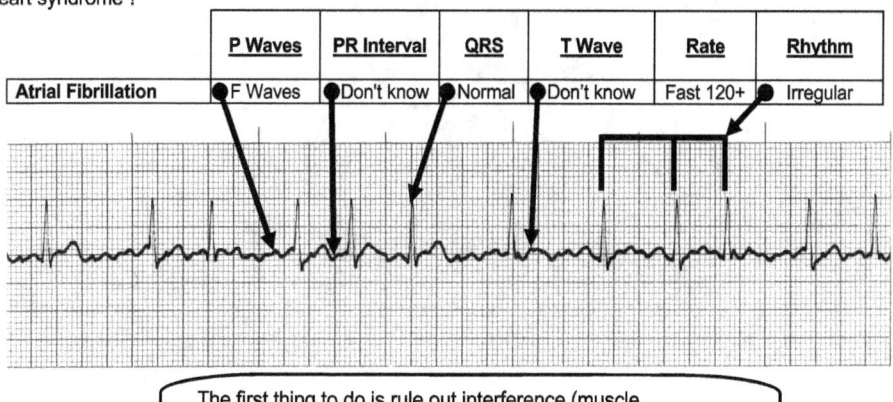

The first thing to do is rule out interference (muscle tremor/electrical). Atrial Fibrillation is an **irregular** rhythm. It is usually a fast rhythm too.

Atrial Flutter

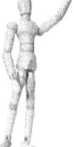

	P Waves	PR Interval	QRS	T Wave	Rate	Rhythm
Sinus Rhythm	Yes	Normal	Normal	Yes	Normal 60-100	Regular
Sinus Tachycardia	Yes	Normal	Normal	Yes	Fast 100-120	Regular
Sinus Bradycardia	Yes	Normal	Normal	Yes	Slow <60	Regular
Sinus Arrhythmia	Yes	Normal	Normal	Yes	Normal	Irregular

	P Waves	PR Interval	QRS	T Wave	Rate	Rhythm
Atrial Tachycardia	Don't know	No	Normal	Don't know	Fast 120-140	Regular
SVT	Don't know	No	Normal	Don't know	Fast 140+	Regular
Atrial Fibrillation	F Waves	Don't know	Normal	Don't know	Fast 120+	Irregular
Atrial Flutter	**Sawtoothed**	**Don't know**	**Normal**	**Don't know**	**Normal or Fast**	**Regular**
Atrial Ectopic (Sinus)	Yes	Yes	Normal	Yes	Any	Irregular
Junctional Ectopic	No	No	Normal	Yes	Any	Irregular

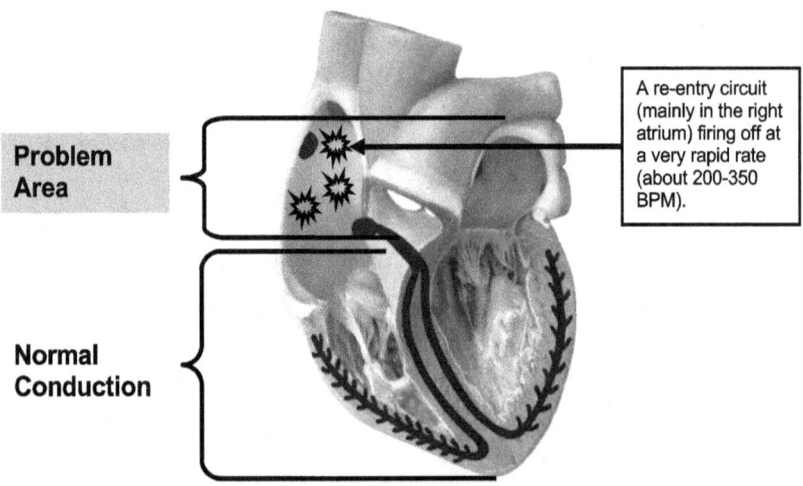

Problem Area

A re-entry circuit (mainly in the right atrium) firing off at a very rapid rate (about 200-350 BPM).

Normal Conduction

Atrial Flutter

This rhythm is fairly distinctive. It can look like a wood saw turned upside down. This one is a **regular** rhythm it also can be normal or fast. It is usually paroxysmal which can last for as long as a few seconds to hours or even days.

On this rhythm, the atria are irritated by one or more cells which cause the atria to go into a rapid re-entry spasm and can produce atrial impulses of about 300 BPM. It is a re-entry circuit supraventricular macroreentry tachycardia (a current that will circle around a large structure) which is confined in the right atrium and usually 90% is in an anticlockwise rotation circuit showing inverted flutter waves best in lead II. The AV node cannot handle these sort of 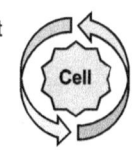 speeds and initiates its self-survival mechanism, so it grabs maybe every 2nd or 4th or more impulses, that comes its way and then passes them down to the ventricles. The normal ratio is 2:1 with a ventricular rate of 150 BPM considered to be indicative of atrial flutter. It is difficult to see if they are P waves or T waves so they are called F (flutter) waves again. The activity looks rather weird and gives off a saw-toothed effect, which makes it quite distinctive as it is a spasm and not fibrillating and quivering. If this does last for a prolonged time, then there is a high chance that it will convert into AF. The ventricular rate is classed as a fraction of the atrial rate so for example, a 2:1 ratio =150 BPM, a 3:1=100 BPM and 4:1=75 BPM.

As the impulse come on a regular basis the rhythm is also a regular one. This is an easy one to confuse with Atrial Fibrillation though; the difference being is that Atrial Flutter is **regular** whilst Atrial Fibrillation is **irregular.**

	P Waves	PR Interval	QRS	T Wave	Rate	Rhythm
Atrial Flutter	Sawtoothed	Don't know	Normal	Don't know	Normal or Fast	Regular

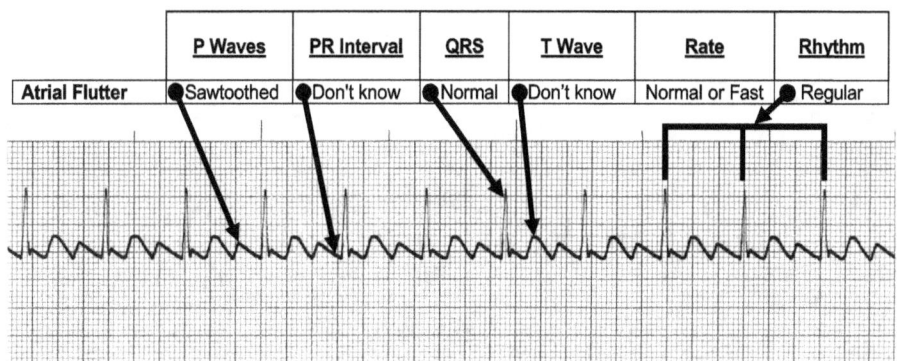

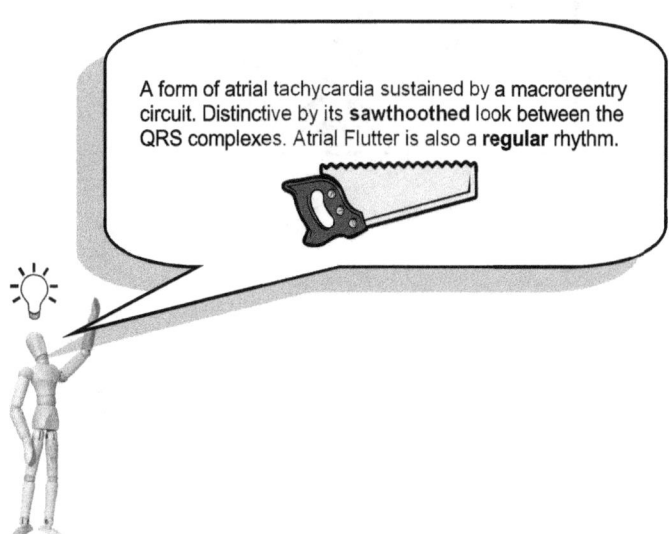

A form of atrial tachycardia sustained by a macroreentry circuit. Distinctive by its **sawthoothed** look between the QRS complexes. Atrial Flutter is also a **regular** rhythm.

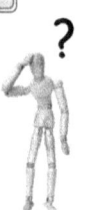

Atrial Ectopic

	P Waves	PR Interval	QRS	T Wave	Rate	Rhythm
Sinus Rhythm	Yes	Normal	Normal	Yes	Normal 60-100	Regular
Sinus Tachycardia	Yes	Normal	Normal	Yes	Fast 100-120	Regular
Sinus Bradycardia	Yes	Normal	Normal	Yes	Slow <60	Regular
Sinus Arrhythmia	Yes	Normal	Normal	Yes	Normal	Irregular

	P Waves	PR Interval	QRS	T Wave	Rate	Rhythm
Atrial Tachycardia	Don't know	No	Normal	Don't know	Fast 120-140	Regular
SVT	Don't know	No	Normal	Don't know	Fast 140+	Regular
Atrial Fibrillation	F Waves	Don't know	Normal	Don't know	Fast 120+	Irregular
Atrial Flutter	Sawtoothed	Don't know	Normal	Don't know	Normal or Fast	Regular
Atrial Ectopic (Sinus)	**Yes**	**Yes**	**Normal**	**Yes**	**Any**	**Irregular**
Junctional Ectopic	No	No	Normal	Yes	Any	Irregular

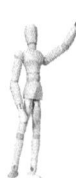

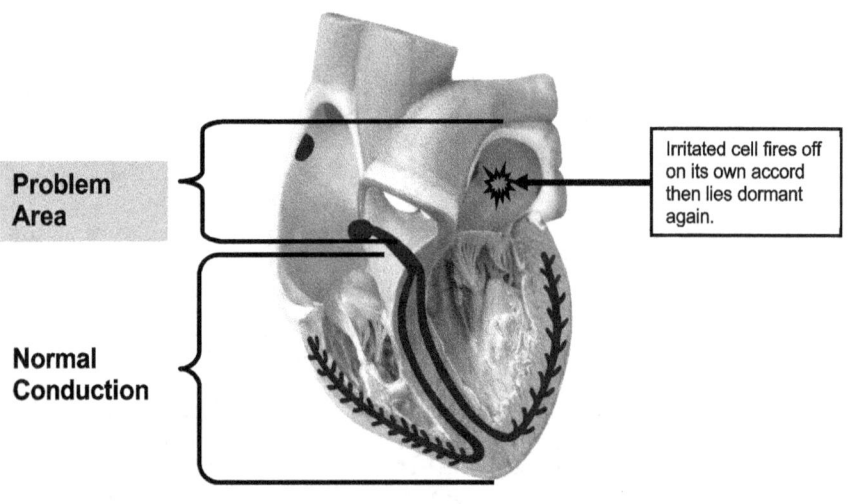

Problem Area

Normal Conduction

Irritated cell fires off on its own accord then lies dormant again.

Atrial Ectopic (AE or PAE)

These are not terribly easy to spot, but if you look carefully you'll get it. The rhythm first appears to be regular then all of a sudden it will be slightly irregular then back to a normal rhythm again. All of the QRS complexes are normal, telling you that it is an atrial problem. As you look you will notice that there are 2 beats in quick succession, there is a longer gap after that then it goes back to normal. Confusing isn't it?

What is happening is that an ectopic focus in the atria is firing off too early. One of the cells is irritated and fires off a rogue beat. The rest then turn round to see what happened which causes a small delay. This is called the compensatory pause. Everything then returns to normal.

So there you have it, a **normal** beat (P, QRS, T) followed by a quick-fire premature beat, followed by a short pause then back to normal again.

Most people who experience these types of ectopics feel nothing at all and are unaware of the ectopic, others are more aware and feel a sort of "thump" as if their heart has stopped every time the ectopic happen. This is because the heart has extra time to fill during the pseudo beat and means that as it has to pump extra blood, this beats with a greater contraction and is more noticeable to some people than others which can be quite uncomfortable and distressing if you are more conscious of them. These are benign beats and are usually made worse by stimulants such as coffee, caffeine, lack of sleep, sudden emotions, various medication, or blood chemical imbalances. They maybe just idiopathic (which is completely unknown). In a normal individual, these are benign and usually a cause which can be removed (stop drinking tea or coffee!).

There are two different types of Atrial Ectopic (or Premature Atrial Ectopic (PAE)), which are sinus and junctional. The sinus type is the easiest it has a P (depending where the focus is, it is usually a different shape the all of the others) wave before the extra QRS, which tells you that it originates from in or near the SA node. The junctional ectopic has no P wave but is explained in the next rhythm.

	P Waves	PR Interval	QRS	T Wave	Rate	Rhythm
Atrial Ectopic (Sinus)	Yes	Yes	Normal	Yes	Normal	Irregular

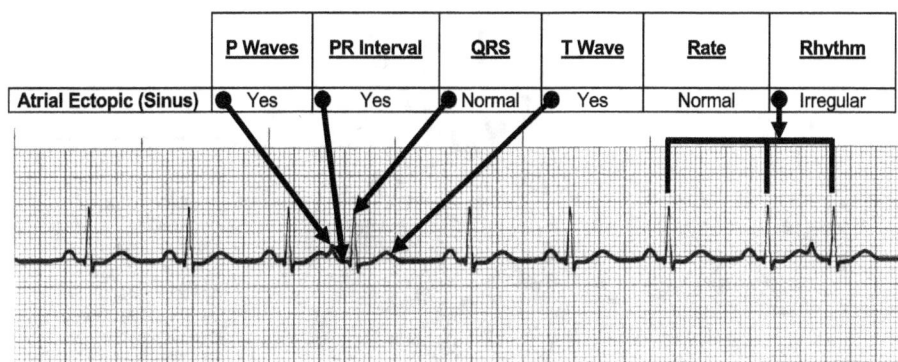

Just a glitch in what seems to be a normal rhythm. There is an extra beat followed by a short pause before returning to normal. Remember that Atrial Ectopics have a **P** wave (often a different shape to the normal P).

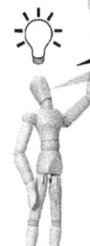

Junctional Ectopic

	P Waves	PR Interval	QRS	T Wave	Rate	Rhythm
Sinus Rhythm	Yes	Normal	Normal	Yes	Normal 60-100	Regular
Sinus Tachycardia	Yes	Normal	Normal	Yes	Fast 100-120	Regular
Sinus Bradycardia	Yes	Normal	Normal	Yes	Slow <60	Regular
Sinus Arrhythmia	Yes	Normal	Normal	Yes	Normal	Irregular

	P Waves	PR Interval	QRS	T Wave	Rate	Rhythm
Atrial Tachycardia	Don't know	No	Normal	Don't know	Fast 120-140	Regular
SVT	Don't know	No	Normal	Don't know	Fast 140+	Regular
Atrial Fibrillation	F Waves	Don't know	Normal	Don't know	Fast 120+	Irregular
Atrial Flutter	Sawtoothed	Don't know	Normal	Don't know	Normal or Fast	Regular
Atrial Ectopic (Sinus)	Yes	Yes	Normal	Yes	Normal	Irregular
Junctional Ectopic	**No**	**No**	**Normal**	**Yes**	**Normal**	**Irregular**

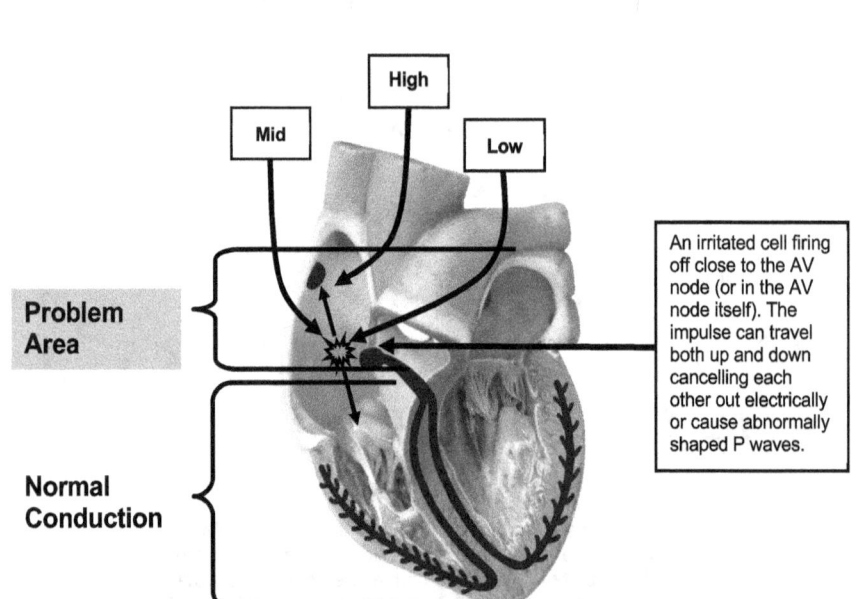

High

Mid

Low

Problem Area

An irritated cell firing off close to the AV node (or in the AV node itself). The impulse can travel both up and down cancelling each other out electrically or cause abnormally shaped P waves.

Normal Conduction

Junctional Ectopic

From the previous rhythm the Atrial Ectopic you will see that this particular rhythm is nearly identical, except for one thing, there are no normal P waves. This tells you that the impulse doesn't originate from the SA node it comes from very close to the AV node. It seems that there is a problem with the SA node so the AV node or cells near the AV node take over as the pacemaker. There are 3 types of junctional ectopic, they can be a high, mid or low AV junctional nodal (it is called nodal because that is the area the impulse comes from, the AV node). The high has the P wave at the start of the "extra" beat but it is inverted (it is upside down, a negative impulse rather than a positive one) before the QRS complex. The mid nodal has **no** P wave before the "extra" beat. Finally, there is the low nodal ectopic, in this one there is a P wave, but it will come **after** the QRS complex or be buried in the T wave (making the T wave more notchy than a normal one). In all three types, the P wave is either not there or abnormal.

The most common type of junctional ectopic and the one we will be concentrating on is the mid-nodal ectopic (the one with no P wave), this means that the impulse from the rogue cell spreads straight up to the atria and straight down to the AV node at the same time so you will find that they both cancel each other out electrically. Everything that produces energy produces a vector i.e. if someone throws three tennis balls towards you and you throw three back then they cancel out each. The same principle applies to electrical signals so distinctively in the mid nodal ectopic, there is **no** P wave at the "extra" beat, or that it could originate from the AV node itself.

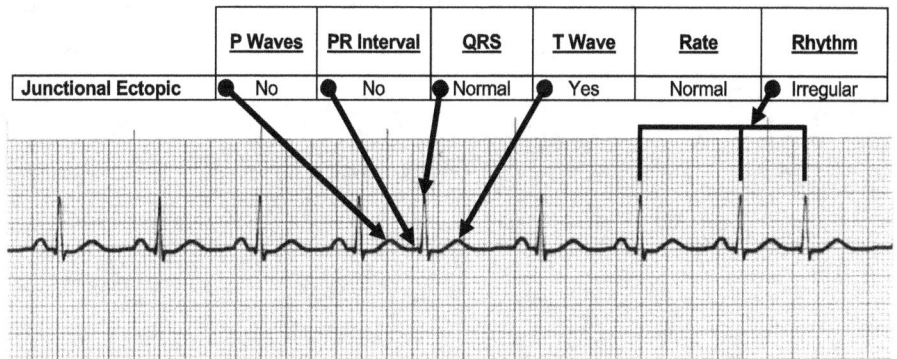

	P Waves	PR Interval	QRS	T Wave	Rate	Rhythm
Junctional Ectopic	No	No	Normal	Yes	Normal	Irregular

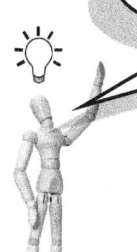

It's a very similar rhythm to the atrial ectopic, but this time there is **no** normal P wave at the extra beat this is because as the irritated impulse spreads up and down at the same time they cancel each other out electrically (a positive signal against a negative signal produces **no** signal). It is usually located from the AV node itself.
Other Junctional ectopics have a late (near the T wave) or inverted P wave depending on the location of the beat.

Ventricular Arrhythmias

Ventricular rhythms are easier to identify than the atrial one because when we look at the initial rhythm we can see that the QRS complex is usually wide and bizarre.

Here is a comparison chart for all Ventricular rhythms.

	P Wave	PR Interval	QRS	T Wave	Rate	Rhythm
Ventricular Ectopic	No	None	Wide/Bizarre	Abnormal	Normal	Irregular
R on T Ectopic	No	None	Wide/Bizarre	Abnormal	Normal	Irregular
Bigeminal Ectopic	No	None	Wide/Bizarre	Abnormal	Slow	Regular
Third Degree Block	Yes	None	Wide/Disassociated	Abnormal	Slow QRS Normal P	Regular
Pacemaker	Maybe	Maybe	Wide/Bizarre with pacing spikes	Abnormal	Normal	Regular
Ventricular Tachycardia	Maybe	None	Wide	No	Very Fast	Regular
Ventricular Fibrillation	Don't know	None	Disorganised	Don't know	Very Fast	Irregular
Asystole	No	None	None	No	None	None
Bundle Branch Block	Maybe	Maybe	Wide/Notched or Jagged	Abnormal	Normal	Regular

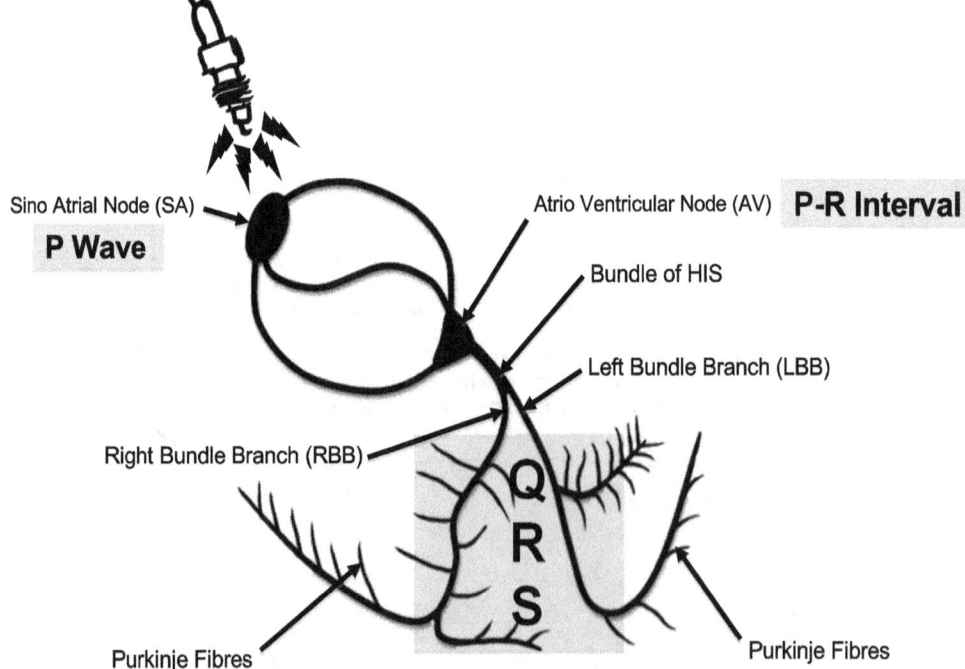

Ventricular rhythms are more life threatening than atrial rhythms.

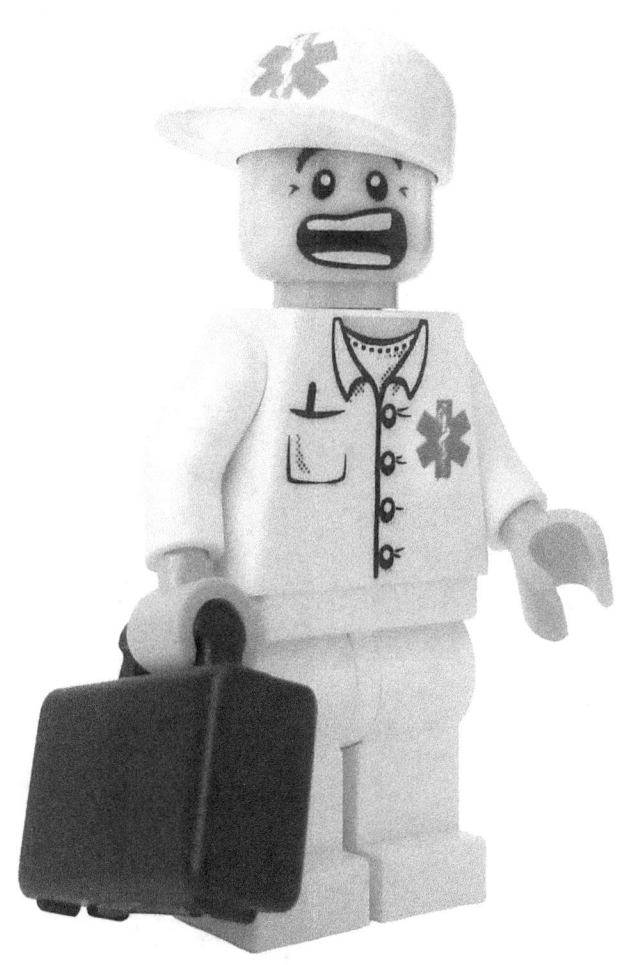

Ventricular Arrhythmias

As you can probably tell, these rhythms have problems that originate in the ventricles, and cause the problems to be seen mainly in the QRS complexes and T waves.

	P Wave	PR Interval	QRS	T Wave	Rate	Rhythm
Ventricular Ectopic	No	None	Wide/Bizarre	Abnormal	Normal	Irregular
R on T Ectopic	No	None	Wide/Bizarre	Abnormal	Normal	Irregular
Bigeminal Ectopic	No	None	Wide/Bizarre	Abnormal	Slow	Regular
Pacemaker	Maybe	Maybe	Wide/Bizarre with pacing spikes	Abnormal	Normal	Regular

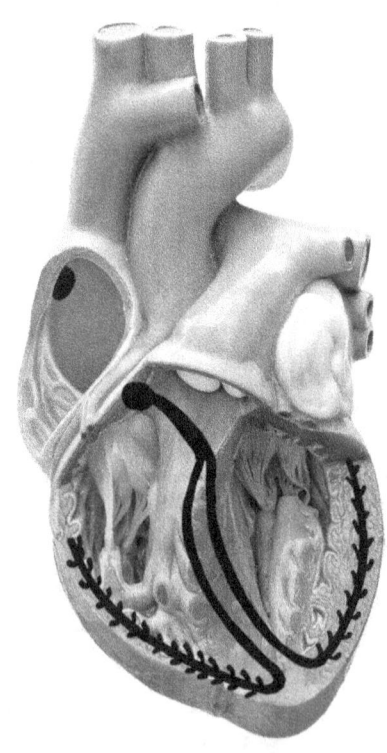

Problem Areas

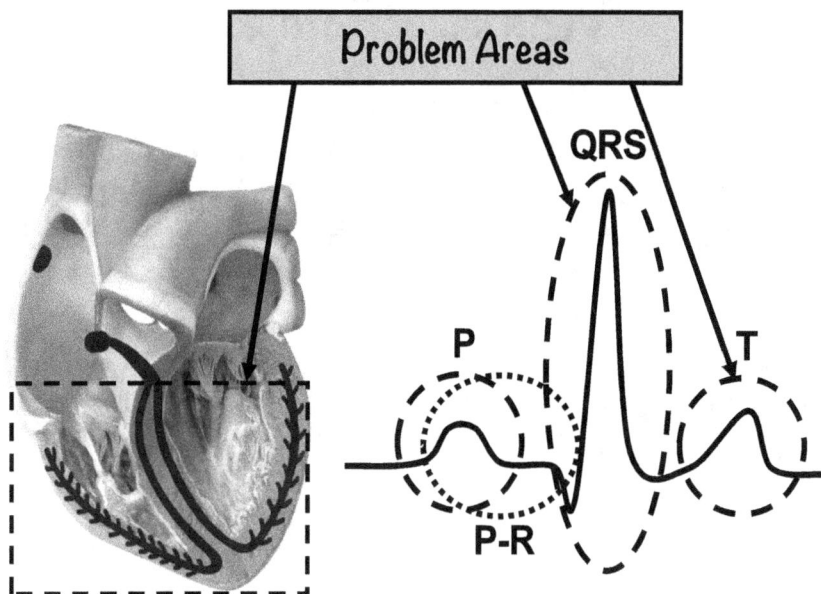

QRS

P

P-R

T

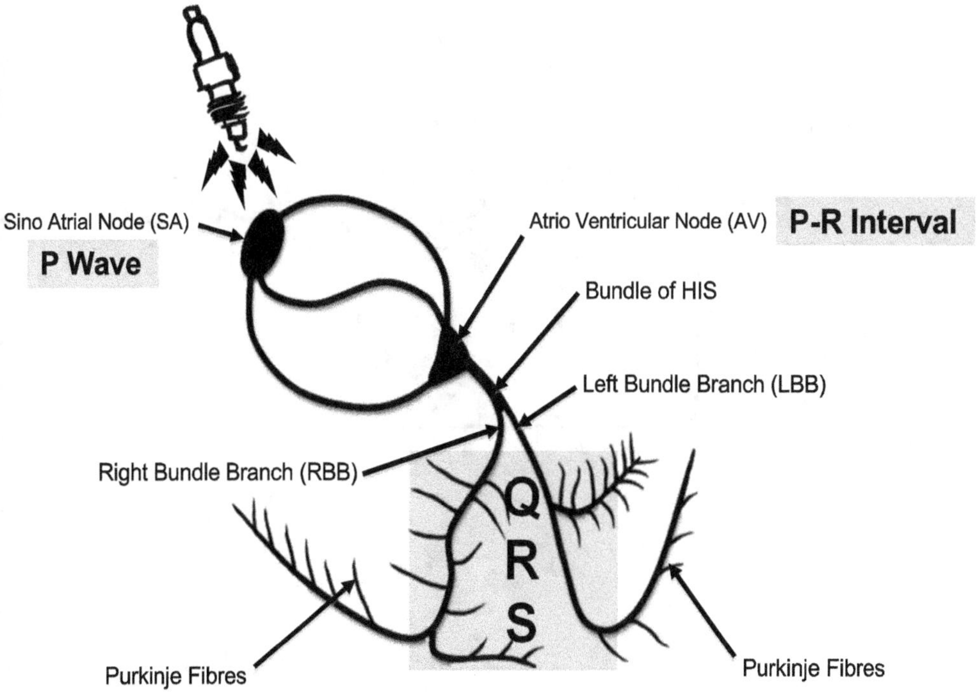

Sino Atrial Node (SA)

P Wave

Atrio Ventricular Node (AV)   **P-R Interval**

Bundle of HIS

Left Bundle Branch (LBB)

Right Bundle Branch (RBB)

Q
R
S

Purkinje Fibres

Purkinje Fibres

Ventricular Ectopic

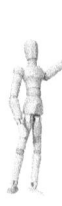

	P Wave	PR Interval	QRS	T Wave	Rate	Rhythm
Ventricular Ectopic	No	None	Wide/Bizarre	Abnormal	Normal	Irregular
R on T Ectopic	No	None	Wide/Bizarre	Abnormal	Normal	Irregular
Bigeminal Ectopic	No	None	Wide/Bizarre	Abnormal	Slow	Regular
Pacemaker	Maybe	Maybe	Wide/Bizarre with pacing spikes	Abnormal	Normal	Regular

Ventricular Tachycardia	Maybe	None	Wide	No	Very Fast	Regular
Ventricular Fibrillation	Don't know	None	Disorganised	Don't know	Very Fast	Irregular
Asystole	No	None	None	No	None	None

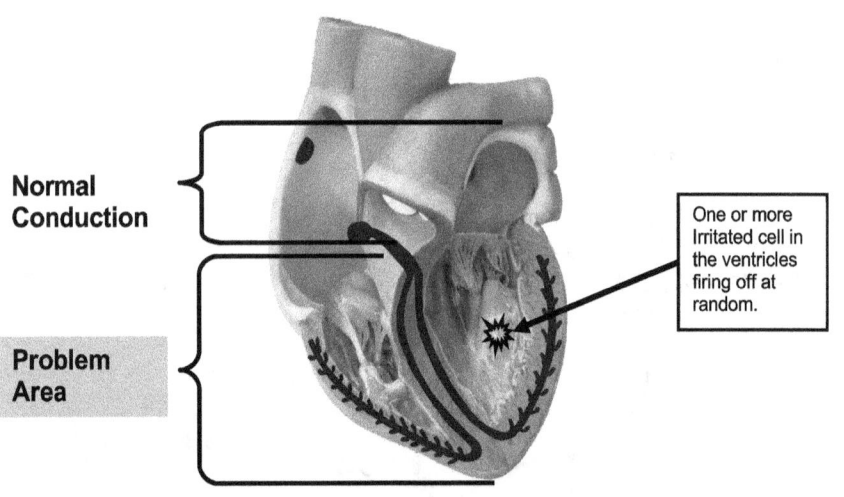

Normal Conduction

Problem Area

One or more Irritated cell in the ventricles firing off at random.

Ventricular Ectopic (VE or PVC)

This one should be nice and easy. It is the first thing that usually strikes you when you look at the rhythm as a whole. This is a relatively common rhythm and it shows up as a really wide and bizarre looking QRS complex. This beat is coming from inside the ventricles in the muscle walls. Again one or a pair of the rogue cells taking control again and causing a blip in the rhythm also sometimes known as a Premature Ventricular Contraction (PVC). It will show up just after the T wave and before the next complex and like the atrial ectopic, there will be a compensatory pause following it.

If you look, you will see that it is greater than three small squares wide, which classes it as wide and bizarre and that it does not follow the determined pathway and could be conducted through slow conducting tissues from within the ventricles, from the Purkinje fibres or from within the ventricular myocardium. The odd one of these ectopic now and again in a normal rhythm is common and doesn't usually present a problem. If they all look the same shape, then they are called unifocal ectopics and they originate from the same focus and take the same route each time. If they are different shapes, they are called multifocal ectopics (they take four different forms). Multifocal ectopics are more of a concern as there is more than one irritated cell firing off in the ventricles and this could cause the ventricles to become hypersensitive and prone to more critical and life threatening rhythms.

Just for a bit of extra knowledge (this can only really be seen in leads V_1 and V_2 in a 12 lead ECG) if the ventricular ectopic has a left bundle branch (or predominantly negative) look, then the rouge beat is from the right ventricle because the impulse is travelling away from the electrode and the delayed activation of the right ventricle. If it has a right bundle branch block (or positive) look then it is from the left ventricle because the impulse travels towards the electrode.

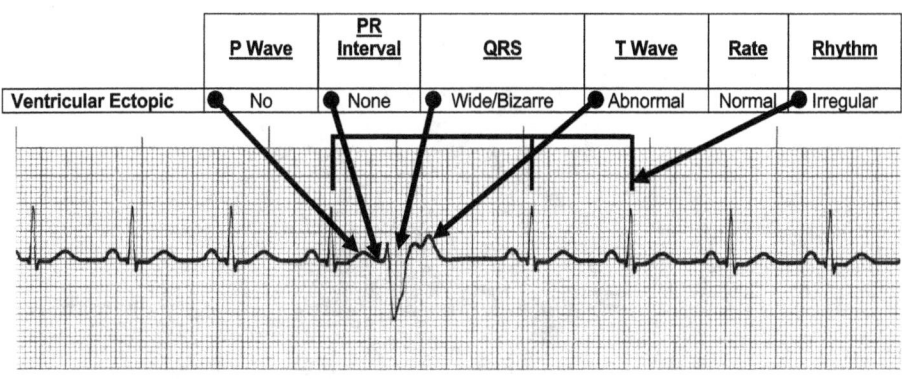

	P Wave	PR Interval	QRS	T Wave	Rate	Rhythm
Ventricular Ectopic	No	None	Wide/Bizarre	Abnormal	Normal	Irregular

More obvious to spot by the wide and bizarre complex, so you can't really miss it! Just make sure that they all look the same (unifocal), they don't come too often (one every couple of minutes is not really a problem) and also that they don't fire off **on** the T wave (see page 28).

R on T Ectopic

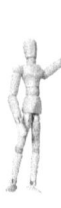

	P Wave	PR Interval	QRS	T Wave	Rate	Rhythm
Ventricular Ectopic	No	None	Wide/Bizarre	Abnormal	Normal	Irregular
R on T Ectopic	No	None	Wide/Bizarre	Abnormal	Normal	Irregular
Bigeminal Ectopic	No	None	Wide/Bizarre	Abnormal	Slow	Regular
Pacemaker	Maybe	Maybe	Wide/Bizarre with pacing spikes	Abnormal	Normal	Regular

	P Wave	PR Interval	QRS	T Wave	Rate	Rhythm
Ventricular Tachycardia	Maybe	None	Wide	No	Very Fast	Regular
Ventricular Fibrillation	Don't know	None	Disorganised	Don't know	Very Fast	Irregular
Asystole	No	None	None	No	None	None

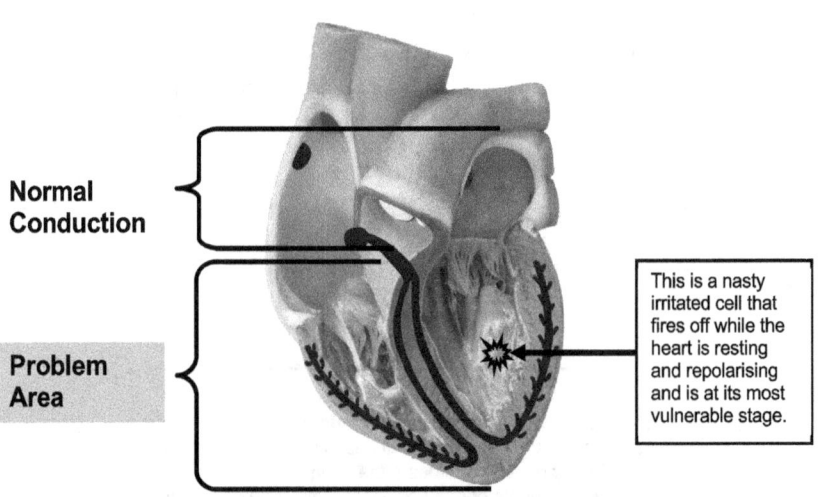

Normal Conduction

Problem Area

This is a nasty irritated cell that fires off while the heart is resting and repolarising and is at its most vulnerable stage.

R on T Ectopic

This is a ventricular ectopic that could turn out to be a nasty one. Let's cast our minds back to a bit in the front of the book (page 28 to be precise) when we talked about the **T** wave. Because of the fact that the heart is repolarising, it is at this time that it is the most vulnerable to any stimulation. This ventricular ectopic decides to fire off right at this particular time, so the **R** wave lands just on the vulnerable crest of the **T** wave itself. If not sorted soon then it could develop into Ventricular Fibrillation as the myocardium is becoming extremely unstable (page 75) and then the real fun starts! Most clinicians will say that the chances of seeing this visually is very slim as the patient will usually present with VF it can be that quick.

It can be a common phenomenon during the first 4 hours of the onset of Myocardial Infarction symptoms but this decreases rapidly with time.

Research shows that this could be the trigger for Sudden Arrhythmic Death (SADS) especially in young adults with conditions like Long QT Syndrome (LQTS), an inherited condition. This means that the T wave and the resting and repolarising phase of the heart takes too long to complete due to a sodium/potassium imbalance and lengthens this important phase (a bit like First Degree Heart Block but with the T wave), so the chances that an adrenaline surge or ectopic has more chance of landing on this prolonged T wave. This can happen at any time during stress, exercise, excitement or even in sleep when the pulse rate naturally slows down. Also some Prescription Only Medicines (POM) or Over The Counter (OTC) medicines such as antibiotics, antihistamines and cold remedies.

Studies have found that diving into cold water extends the QT and this may be a cause for the unexplained sudden drowning phenomenon, especially in good swimmers.

	P Wave	PR Interval	QRS	T Wave	Rate	Rhythm
R on T Ectopic	No	None	Wide/Bizarre	Abnormal	Normal	Irregular

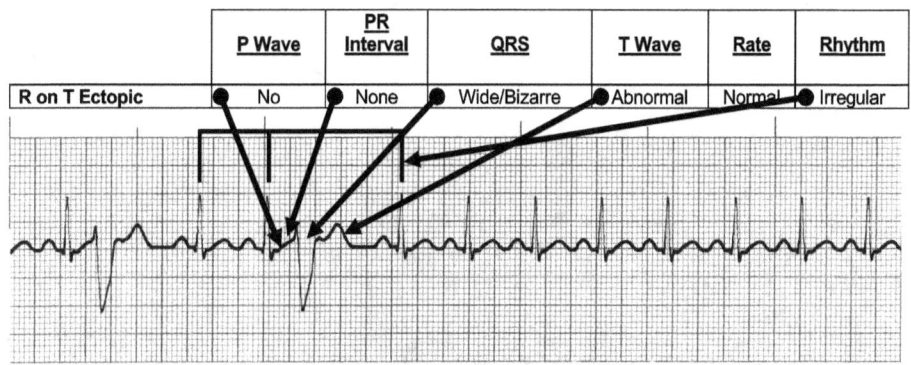

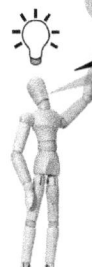

Looks just like a normal Ventricular Ectopic but the R wave fires **ON** the vulnerable phase of the T wave. Watch out for this one as it could send the rhythm into Ventricular Fibrillation (VF) very quickly!

Bigeminy

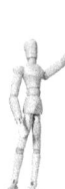

	P Wave	PR Interval	QRS	T Wave	Rate	Rhythm
Ventricular Ectopic	No	None	Wide/Bizarre	Abnormal	Normal	Irregular
R on T Ectopic	No	None	Wide/Bizarre	Abnormal	Normal	Irregular
Bigeminal Ectopic	**No**	**None**	**Wide/Bizarre**	**Abnormal**	**Slow**	**Regular**
Pacemaker	Maybe	Maybe	Wide/Bizarre with pacing spikes	Abnormal	Normal	Regular

	P Wave	PR Interval	QRS	T Wave	Rate	Rhythm
Ventricular Tachycardia	Maybe	None	Wide	No	Very Fast	Regular
Ventricular Fibrillation	Don't know	None	Disorganised	Don't know	Very Fast	Irregular
Asystole	No	None	None	No	None	None

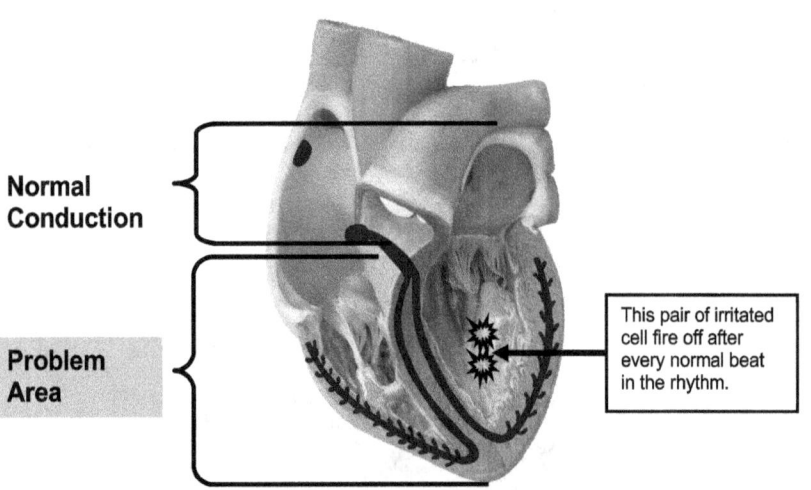

Normal Conduction

Problem Area

This pair of irritated cell fire off after every normal beat in the rhythm.

Bigeminy (BGY)

This is a regular rhythm. You will see that the underlying rhythm is usually Sinus Rhythm, but after every normal beat is a ventricular ectopic and this regularly alternates between a normal and an abnormal beat. It is also usually a constant one but it can come and go (paroxysmal) with some people experiencing some shortness of breath or tiredness during the episode. Bi-geminy means every **two**- beats, like bi-focal glasses, means **two**-focusing lenses or bi-cycle means **two**-wheeled cycle. If it was trigeminy, this would be **two** normal beats to **one** ectopic (every three e.g. tri-angle).

If you take this person's pulse without looking at the monitor, you may think that this is probably just a sinus bradycardia rate, but if you look at the screen at the same time as taking the pulse you will only be able to feel the normal beats giving the impression initially of a bradycardic pulse. They may also feel faint or lightheaded especially when standing.

A true Bigeminy will have a compensatory pause after each normal pulse and could be sustained or paroxysmal (comes and goes away).

Under normal circumstances, the rapid strength of the normal impulse will suppress any rouge cell impulse from above so most will not show up. However, the if the ectopic focus fires within the ventricles, it will depolarise the ventricles directly and bypass the HIS and the Purkinje system. Apart from the obvious possible bradycardia, it will put the beating of the ventricles out of sync. The is some evidence that the Bigeminy is from a fixed re-entry of ectopics which form the Bigeminal rhythm (and, of course, the trigeminal too).

	P Wave	PR Interval	QRS	T Wave	Rate	Rhythm
Bigeminal Ectopic	● No	● None	● Wide/Bizarre	● Abnormal	Slow	● Regular

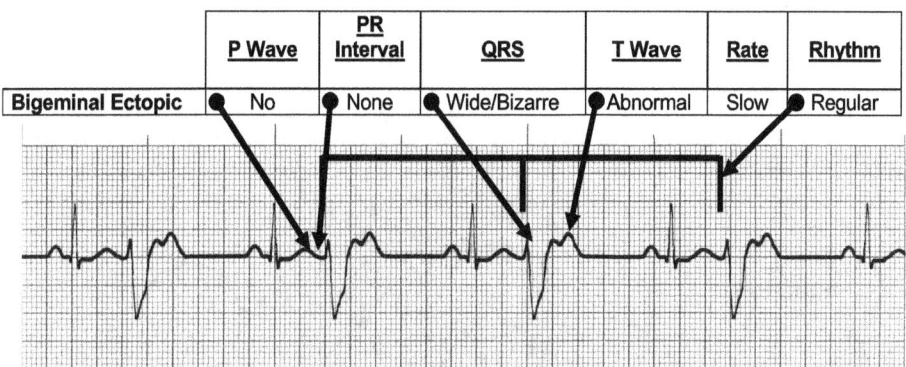

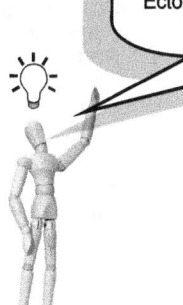

It is called Bigeminy because it is every other beat (bi=2). If you take someone's pulse before seeing this one, you may think that it is Bradycardia, as you will not be able to feel the Ectopic.

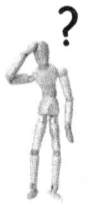

Pacemaker

	P Wave	PR Interval	QRS	T Wave	Rate	Rhythm
Ventricular Ectopic	No	None	Wide/Bizarre	Abnormal	Normal	Irregular
R on T Ectopic	No	None	Wide/Bizarre	Abnormal	Normal	Irregular
Bigeminal Ectopic	No	None	Wide/Bizarre	Abnormal	Slow	Regular
Pacemaker	Maybe	Maybe	Wide/Bizarre with pacing spikes	Abnormal	Normal	Regular
Ventricular Tachycardia	Maybe	None	Wide	No	Very Fast	Regular
Ventricular Fibrillation	Don't know	None	Disorganised	Don't know	Very Fast	Irregular
Asystole	No	None	None	No	None	None

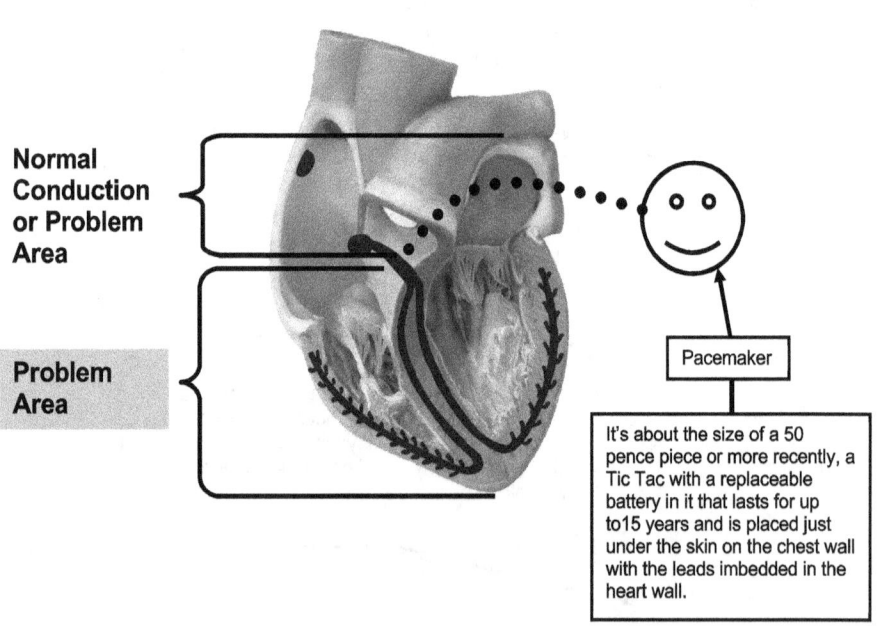

Normal Conduction or Problem Area

Problem Area

Pacemaker

It's about the size of a 50 pence piece or more recently, a Tic Tac with a replaceable battery in it that lasts for up to15 years and is placed just under the skin on the chest wall with the leads imbedded in the heart wall.

Pacemaker

This is one that can catch you out, but this is not so much a problem rhythm as an old problem with new bionic super-duper high-tech gadgetry to sort it. Pacemakers are a common cure for someone with a third degree heart block (page 87) if the heart has congenital problems with the heart rate going too slow or too fast or there is damage to the normal conductive pathway from a heart attack or disease. There are usually two types of pacemaker one that paces all the time and the other that is set to work on demand when the heart rate goes too low or too high. Because the AV node is having a few (well a lot really) problems then an artificial pacemaker has been implanted to take control of the ventricles and pace them into a normal rhythm. A person with one of these can if it is working ok, lead a fairly normal lifestyle. Technology is so advanced that the pacemaker functions can be changed externally without the need for extra surgery.

The QRS complexes look wide and bizarre, so it looks like a third degree heart block or a Bundle Branch Block (page 89). The rhythm should be regular unless there is a problem. The giveaway for this one is a pacing spike just before or in the QRS complex. The ventricles cannot produce a straight line on an ECG this is the artificial conduction of the pacemaker. If the pacemaker is working ok, then the wide and bizarre QRS complexes aren't a problem. Sometimes you may see P waves or you may not as the SA node could still be working. Some of the most up to date pacemakers do not show prominent or very subtle pacing spikes on the ECG but the newer ECG monitors can detect this subtlety and can print arrows on the rhythm strip but the best person to ask about their pacemaker is the patient. To note there will almost certainly be T wave abnormalities.

It is also worth noting that there are pacemakers used which pace the atria and not just the ventricles or there are ones that can even pace both atria and ventricles (dual chamber). These are not as common as the ventricular pacemaker, so as not to confuse you too much we will concentrate on the one that you are more likely to come across.

	P Wave	PR Interval	QRS	T Wave	Rate	Rhythm
Pacemaker	Maybe	Maybe	Wide/Bizarre with pacing spikes	Abnormal	Normal	Regular

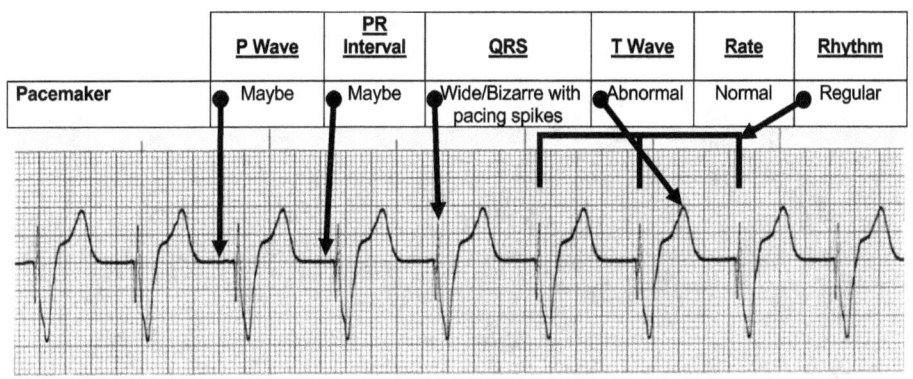

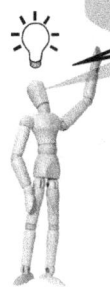

Looks at first glance to be 3rd Degree Heart Block, but the **ventricular** pacing spikes give you a clue. Also the rate is **normal** if the pacemaker is working ok whereas 3rd Degree is normally a **very slow** one.

The Oh Dear! Section

This section gives you some of the most obvious rhythms you will see and also the most life threatening of all rhythms. These are the ones that you should be able to recognise very quickly as you haven't got much time to sit and admire them. The normal reaction to seeing these rhythms is Oh dear! (or something similar! hence the title of this section) as you quickly realise what they are.

	P Wave	PR Interval	QRS	T Wave	Rate	Rhythm
Ventricular Tachycardia	Maybe	None	Wide	No	Very Fast	Regular
Ventricular Fibrillation	Don't know	None	Disorganised	Don't know	Very Fast	Irregular
Asystole	No	None	None	No	None	None

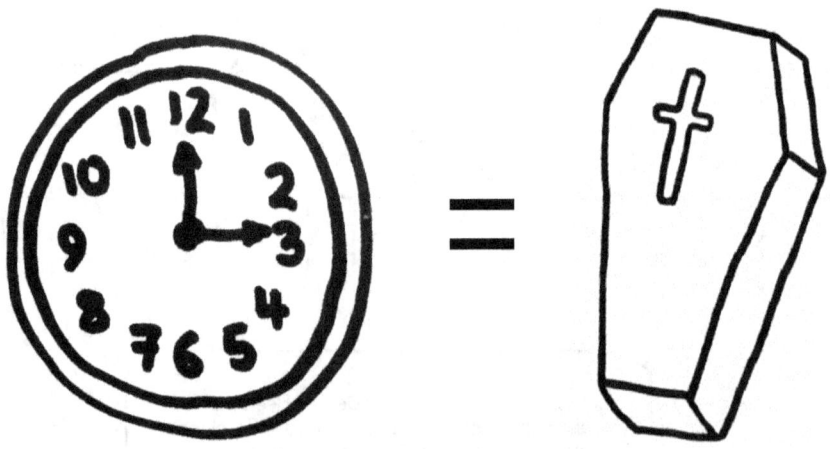

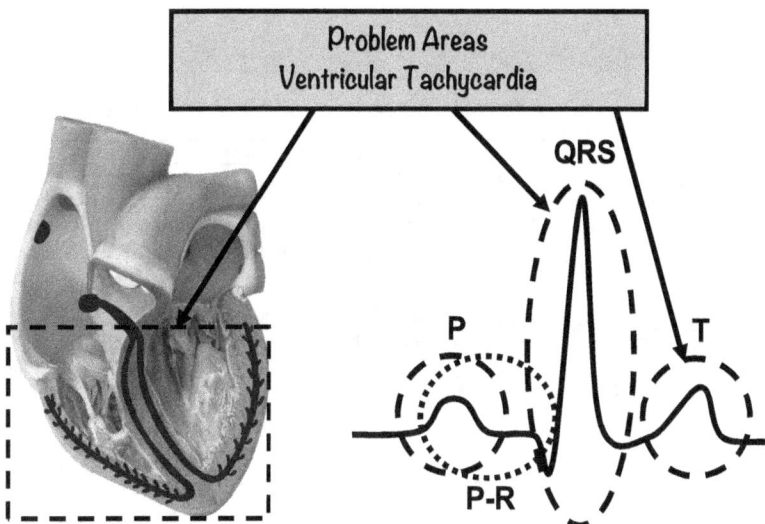

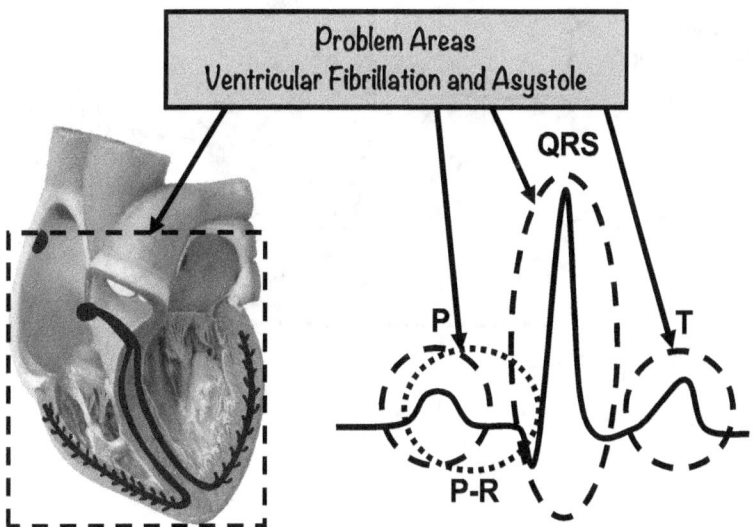

Ventricular Tachycardia

	P Wave	PR Interval	QRS	T Wave	Rate	Rhythm
Ventricular Ectopic	No	None	Wide/Bizarre	Abnormal	Normal	Irregular
R on T Ectopic	No	None	Wide/Bizarre	Abnormal	Normal	Irregular
Bigeminal Ectopic	No	None	Wide/Bizarre	Abnormal	Slow	Regular
Pacemaker	Maybe	Maybe	Wide/Bizarre with pacing spikes	Abnormal	Normal	Regular

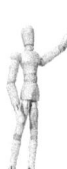

Ventricular Tachycardia	Maybe	None	Wide	No	Very Fast	Regular
Ventricular Fibrillation	Don't know	None	Disorganised	Don't know	Very Fast	Irregular
Asystole	No	None	None	No	None	None

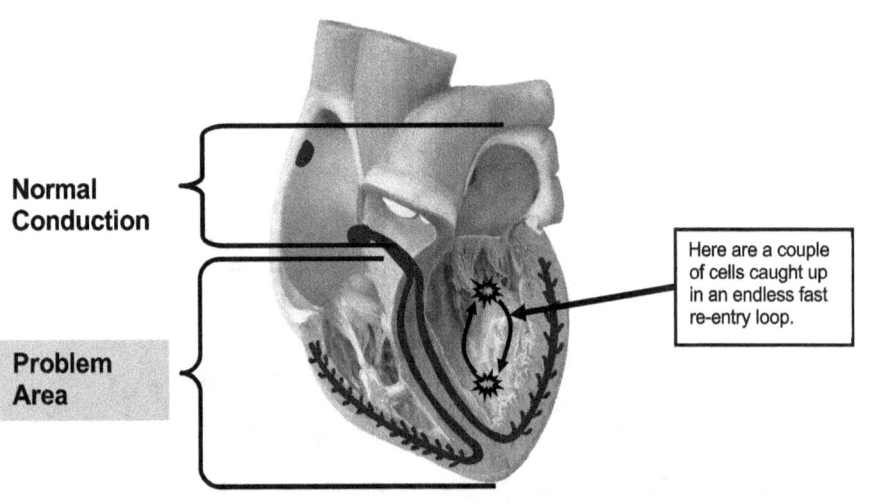

Normal Conduction

Problem Area

Here are a couple of cells caught up in an endless fast re-entry loop.

Ventricular Tachycardia (VT)

This is classed in your "oh dear" section. Another couple of hypersensitive rogue cells in the ventricles usually near or in either on the Bundle Branches or just as an idiopathic cause but it can come from anywhere in the myocardium as there are infinite locations from where it can start from and there will be no fixed waveform pattern. The cells discharge at a fast rate and gets stuck in an indefinite re-entry loop with themselves from which they can't break free. The re-entry impulse just keeps getting faster and faster. Because it comes from the ventricles, you will see that QRS complex will be wide and bizarre (as the conduction is not through the normal conductive pathway. The heart rate itself can be as slow as over 100 BPM or as fast as >200 BPM (VT is defined as more than three consecutive ventricular complexes >100 BPM), but no matter what speed, it still can't break free from this indefinite loop without physical or medicated interventions. The problem is this fast ventricular rate cannot be tolerated by the heart for too long and being a muscle; the heart will eventually get tired and give up as it also is starving itself of oxygen because of the standstill. Because of the fast rate, the ventricles cannot fill to properly causing fatigue and if not careful can induce Ventricular Fibrillation (Page 75), which of course will give you a bigger problem!

You might not find a pulse or blood pressure on this person because the ventricles are beating so fast that they have not got time to fill up sufficiently and the patient will quickly be losing consciousness.

Meanwhile, the atria unaware of the problem downstairs, still continue to beat at a normal rate. If you look closely enough you might just see small P waves buried in various points of the complex. You will also find that this rhythm is a very **slightly** irregular one as opposed to SVT, which is regular, but you will have to look very closely to see this. You may get a normal beat in amongst the rhythm which is called a capture or fusion beat as the normal atrial and ventricular actions finally catch up with each other (these beats can actually terminate paroxysmal VT). This is common for someone with heart disease or a cardiomyopathy and an increased chance of this rhythm after having an MI.

When I see this rhythm, it always reminds me of a row of deckchairs stacked up!

The only way to rectify this is if they have no pulse and are unconscious, is to attempt to "convert" this rhythm into a normal rhythm using defibrillation and darn good CPR as it is now a cardiac arrest.

To tell if this tachycardia comes from the right or the left ventricle then look in lead II. If it is a positive QRS complex, then it will come from the right ventricle as the impulse is going towards the electrode. Therefore, if it a negative complex then it will come from the left ventricle as the impulse moves away from the electrode.

	P Wave	PR Interval	QRS	T Wave	Rate	Rhythm
Ventricular Tachycardia	Maybe	None	Wide	No	Very Fast	Regular

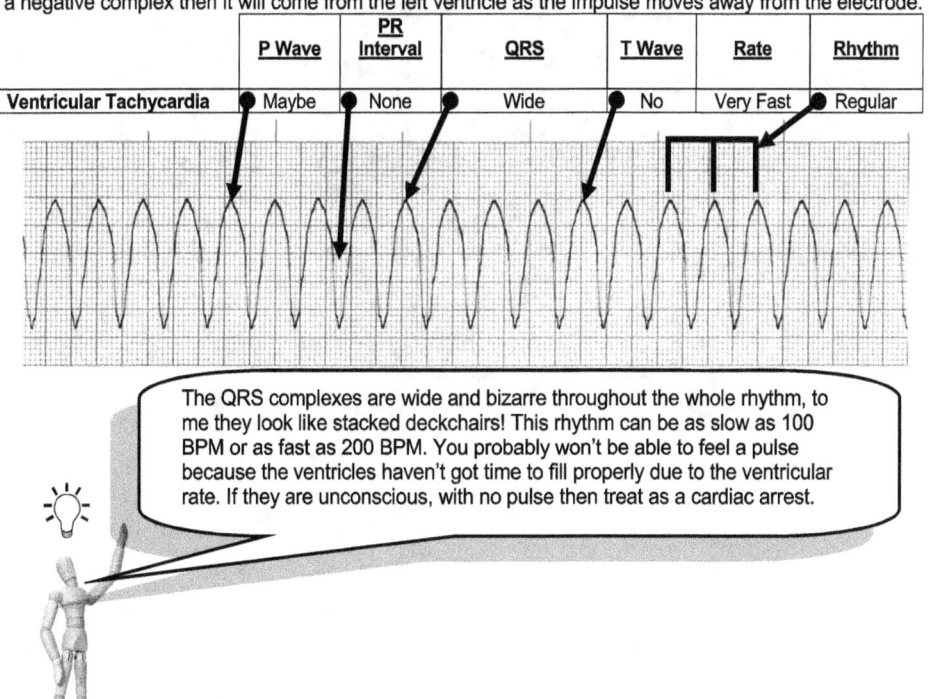

The QRS complexes are wide and bizarre throughout the whole rhythm, to me they look like stacked deckchairs! This rhythm can be as slow as 100 BPM or as fast as 200 BPM. You probably won't be able to feel a pulse because the ventricles haven't got time to fill properly due to the ventricular rate. If they are unconscious, with no pulse then treat as a cardiac arrest.

Ventricular Fibrillation

	P Wave	PR Interval	QRS	T Wave	Rate	Rhythm
Ventricular Ectopic	No	None	Wide/Bizarre	Abnormal	Normal	Irregular
R on T Ectopic	No	None	Wide/Bizarre	Abnormal	Normal	Irregular
Bigeminal Ectopic	No	None	Wide/Bizarre	Abnormal	Slow	Regular
Pacemaker	Maybe	Maybe	Wide/Bizarre with pacing spikes	Abnormal	Normal	Regular

	P Wave	PR Interval	QRS	T Wave	Rate	Rhythm
Ventricular Tachycardia	Maybe	None	Wide	No	Very Fast	Regular
Ventricular Fibrillation	Don't know	None	Disorganised	Don't know	Very Fast	Irregular
Asystole	No	None	None	No	None	None

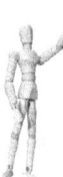

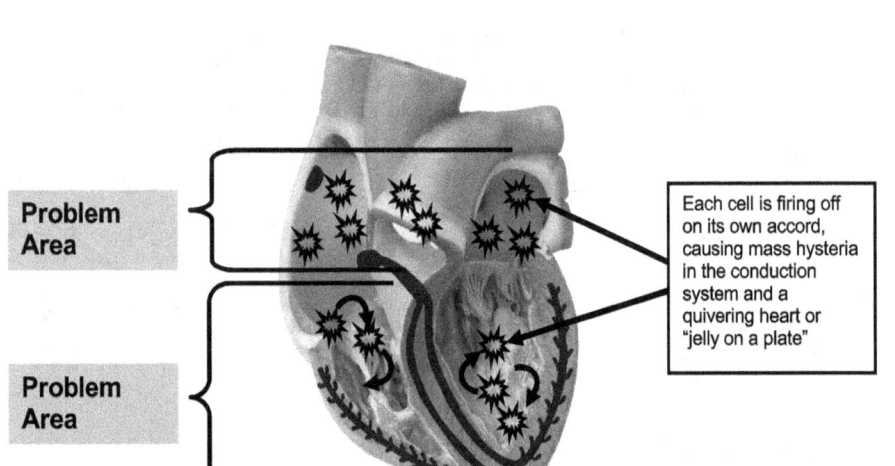

Problem Area

Problem Area

Each cell is firing off on its own accord, causing mass hysteria in the conduction system and a quivering heart or "jelly on a plate"

Ventricular Fibrillation (VF)

Another of the Oh dear! ones. This is mass hysteria in the heart's electrical system. If you look at what is happening to the atria in the Atrial Fibrillation rhythm, then also apply that to the ventricles as well. You will see that all the heart is doing is sitting there like quivering jelly on a plate and is not beating at all, with a loss of coordinated contraction of the myocytes (muscle cells) around the myocardium. The rhythm shows up as a completely uncoordinated and disorganised one and is an easy one to recognise. This is now cardiac arrest time! However, stop and think first. Before you start to panic, **CHECK YOUR PATIENT**. If they are sitting there talking to you then you may just have a loose lead or faulty electrode! Someone in ventricular fibrillation (or VF) will be unconscious; there will be no pulse and the heart is not beating, they are clinically dead. The only way to possibly reverse this is by early defibrillation and good CPR. At first, the VF will appear to be very distinctively wavy (as below) and is known as "coarse VF". If left too long then the electrical activity just becomes less and less and becomes "fine VF", looking like small ripples rather than waves which get weaker as the oxygen is depleted until you have no electrical activity at all and then you have Asystole or as it is commonly known especially in the movies as, "flatline" (see the next rhythm). However, the newer theory about VF is that it is not as uncoordinated as first thought. Look again at the rhythm and you will see that it seems to create a spiral of activity and is thought to be a result of meandering spiral waves, scroll waves or rotors. Another hypothesis is that it could be small multiple daughter wavelets meandering around or off the mother wave. Looking at these theories would seem to make sense as to why VF is not as "uncoordinated" as we first thought. What really amazes me is that the first possible debateable mention about of ventricular fibrillation dates as far back as circa 1500 BC and referred to in the Papyrus Ebers manuscript. However, more recently with the aid of modern imaging scanners, more is being discovered about this lethal rhythm. Whichever way you look at it and how pretty and amazing it may be, prompt defibrillation and if needed, good CPR is the only answer to terminating the arrhythmia and allowing the SA node to take control again.
Just to add a spanner to the works and if you want to do some homework (it is up to you as I am not going to go into detail), there is a rhythm called Torsade De Pointes (French for twisting on a point), which looks similar but your patient will be conscious. That is why it is important to know the difference between the two!

	P Wave	PR Interval	QRS	T Wave	Rate	Rhythm
Ventricular Fibrillation	Don't know	None	Disorganised	Don't know	Very Fast	Irregular

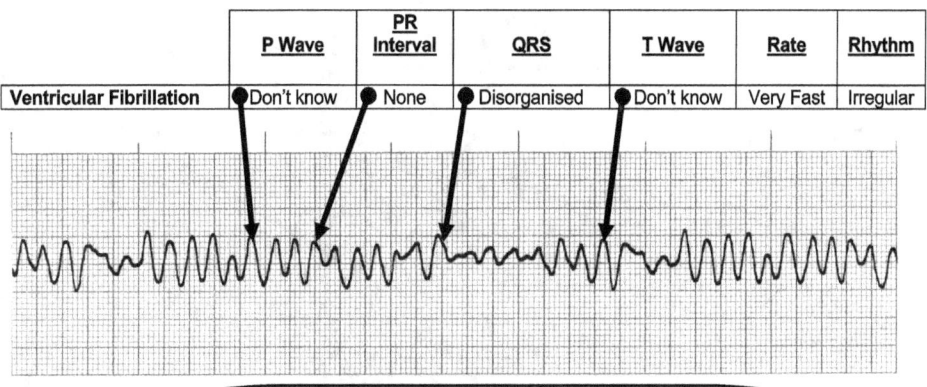

If this is Ventricular Fibrillation, then you won't be able to mistake. It is just a continuous squiggly line but the patient will be unconscious and with no pulse. but before you panic, check to see if any of the leads or electrodes have come astray!

Asystole

	P Wave	PR Interval	QRS	T Wave	Rate	Rhythm
Ventricular Ectopic	No	None	Wide/Bizarre	Abnormal	Normal	Irregular
R on T Ectopic	No	None	Wide/Bizarre	Abnormal	Normal	Irregular
Bigeminal Ectopic	No	None	Wide/Bizarre	Abnormal	Slow	Regular
Pacemaker	Maybe	Maybe	Wide/Bizarre with pacing spikes	Abnormal	Normal	Regular

	P Wave	PR Interval	QRS	T Wave	Rate	Rhythm
Ventricular Tachycardia	Maybe	None	Wide	No	Very Fast	Regular
Ventricular Fibrillation	Don't know	None	Disorganised	Don't know	Very Fast	Irregular
Asystole	**No**	**None**	**None**	**No**	**None**	**None**

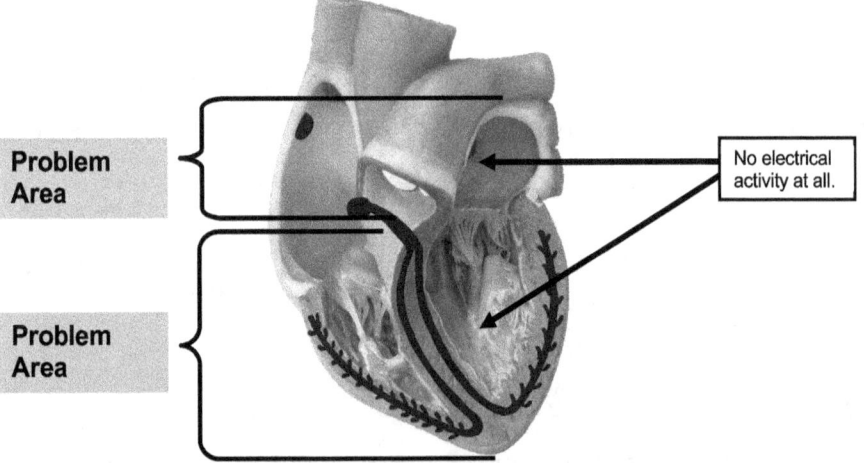

Problem Area

Problem Area

No electrical activity at all.

Asystole (ASY)

This is yet another "Oh Dear!" rhythm. You will probably have heard this on television and films as "flatline". In this rhythm there is no electrical activity of the heart, there is no pulse as the heart has stopped beating. This person is now in cardiac arrest and is clinically dead.

The line you see will not be perfectly straight; if you do something might not be connected properly on your machine so check the connections both on the ECG monitor and the patient before you diagnose this one! Some of the older ECG monitors showed a solid line when the patient was not connected giving you the appearance of Asystole, but most modern monitors will show a broken line so that you know that your patient is not connected to avoid this, it does help!

You may actually see one or two wide and bizarre complexes cropping up now and again on the screen this is usually the dying heart syndrome (idioventricular) and mustn't be confused with a sustained rhythm. These will be seen way too far between each other to be a rhythm.

Ventricular Fibrillation mentioned earlier, if left long enough will eventually go into Asystole and if not treated promptly the electrical impulse gets weaker and weaker until there isn't one, "flatline".

You will also find that kids (bless 'em) due to their high metabolic rate and high use of oxygen and glucose are very prone to go quickly into Asystole during a cardiac arrest. It is rare (or very lucky!) if you see them in VF.

There is not a lot you can do for this rhythm except CPR and drug therapy. Contrary to television and film beliefs you cannot defibrillate someone in this rhythm as you need to have an electrical signal to convert into a normal rhythm and there is **no** electrical activity in this rhythm. Automatic External Defibrillators (AEDs) are becoming more common in the community and use clever software and will not shock in this rhythm during a cardiac arrest and prove to be of no benefit and would delay quality CPR, which is what saves lives.

	P Wave	PR Interval	QRS	T Wave	Rate	Rhythm
Asystole	No	None	None	No	None	None

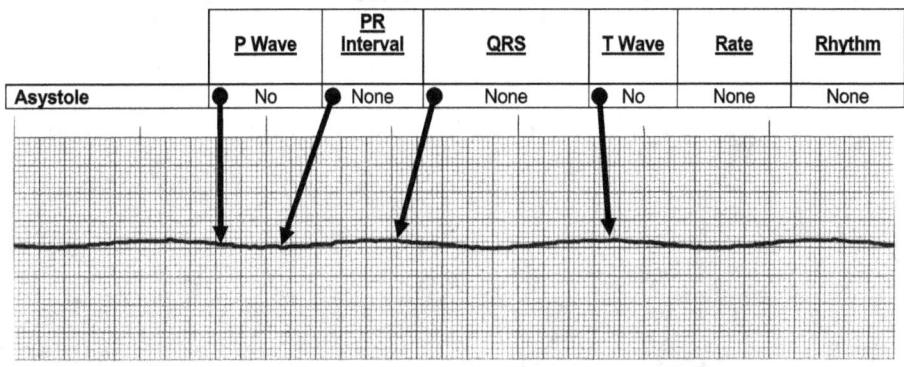

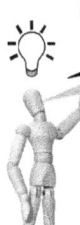

This is commonly known as "flatline", but this is rarely a true flat line. If it is then check the lead connections between the patient and the monitor and see if one or more of the leads or electrodes have slipped off.

Heart Blocks

These all have a problem in and around the AV node area, which causes problems from the PR interval onwards (or should I say downwards!). This affects mainly the PR interval and the rhythm of the ECG.

This is the case in the first three of our less serious rhythms, but the last two are considered more serious as the QRS complexes are affected.

	P Waves	PR Interval	QRS	T Wave	Rate	Rhythm
First Degree Heart Block	Yes	Long	Normal	Yes	Normal	Regular
Second Degree Type One	Yes	Lengthens	Normal	Not Always	Normal	Regularly Irregular
Second Degree Type Two	Yes	Sometimes	Normal	Not Always	Normal	Regular
Third Degree Heart Block	Yes	None	Wide/ Disassociated	Abnormal	Slow QRS Normal P	Regular
Bundle Branch Block	Maybe	Maybe	Wide/Notched Or Jagged	Abnormal	Normal	Regular

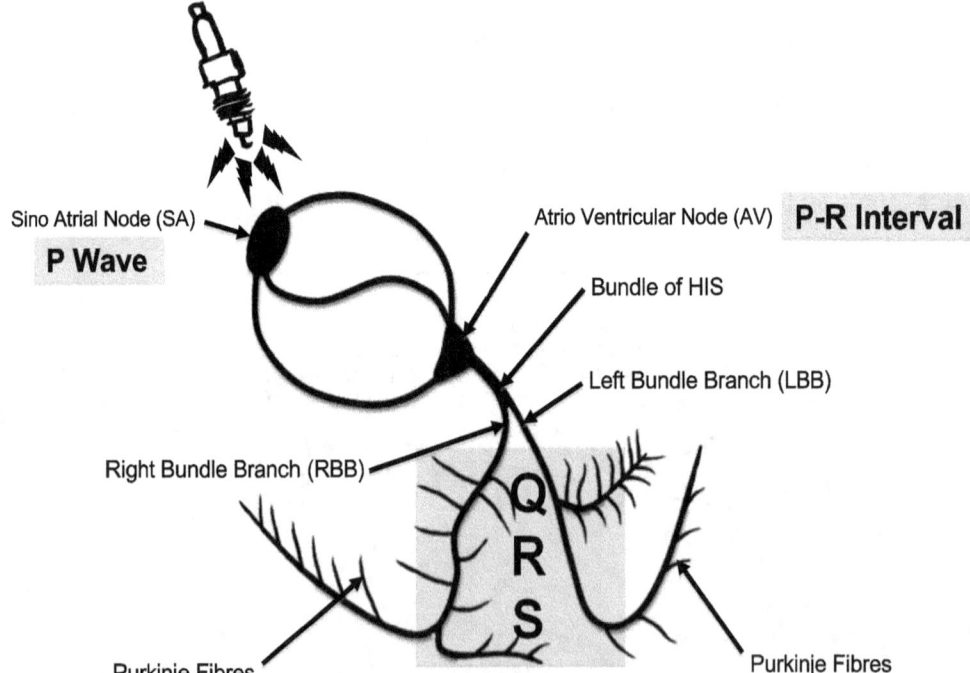

Sino Atrial Node (SA)

P Wave

Atrio Ventricular Node (AV)   **P-R Interval**

Bundle of HIS

Left Bundle Branch (LBB)

Right Bundle Branch (RBB)

Q R S

Purkinje Fibres

Purkinje Fibres

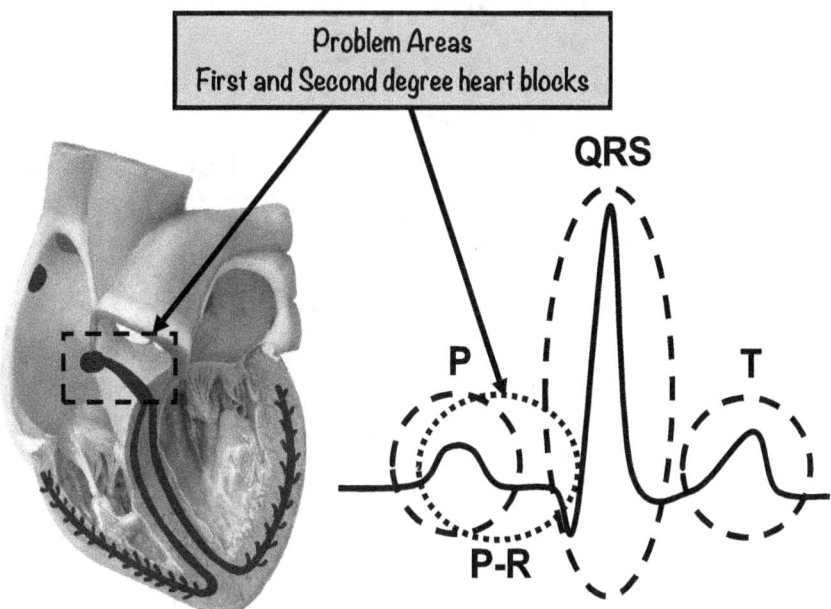

Problem Areas
First and Second degree heart blocks

QRS

P

T

P-R

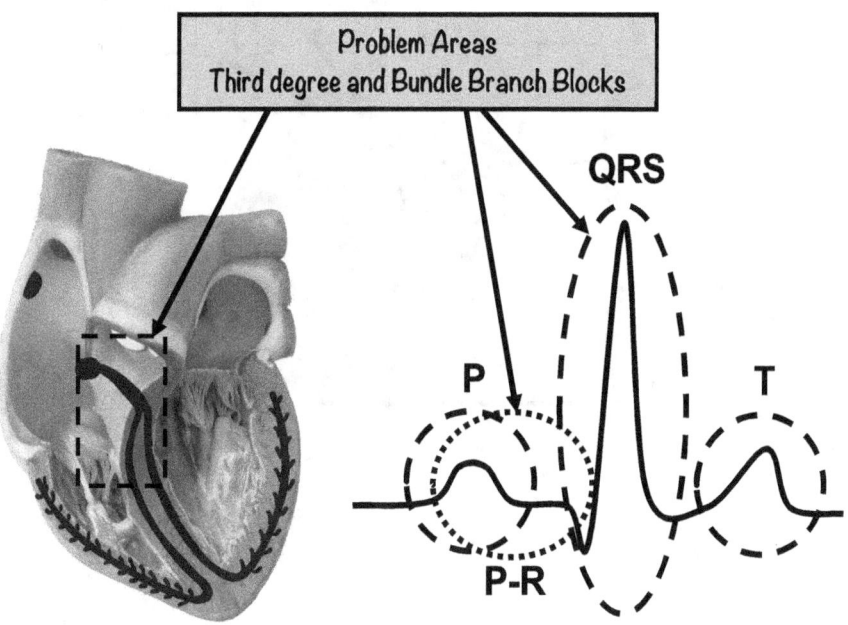

Problem Areas
Third degree and Bundle Branch Blocks

QRS

P

T

P-R

First Degree Heart Block

	P Waves	PR Interval	QRS	T Wave	Rate	Rhythm
First Degree Heart Block	Yes	Long	Normal	Yes	Normal	Regular
Second Degree Type One	Yes	Lengthens	Normal	Not Always	Normal	Regularly Irregular
Second Degree Type Two	Yes	Sometimes	Normal	Not Always	Normal	Regular
Third Degree Heart Block	Yes	None	Wide/ Disassociated	Abnormal	Slow QRS Normal P	Regular
Bundle Branch Block	Maybe	Maybe	Wide/Notched Or Jagged	Abnormal	Normal	Regular

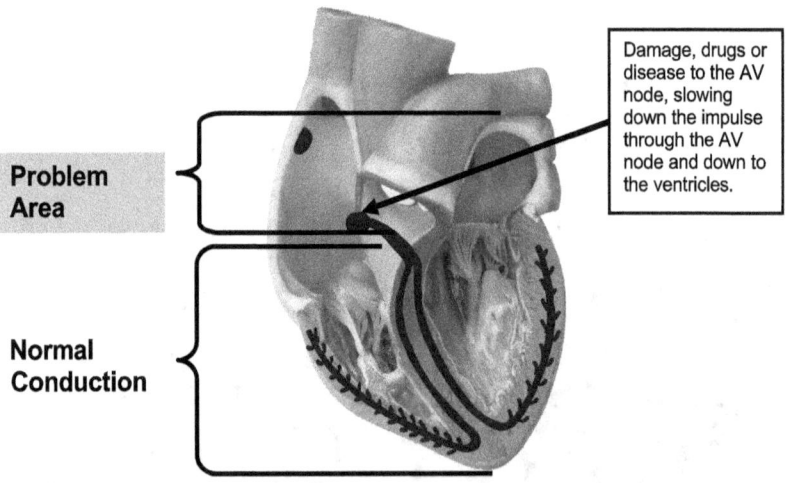

Problem Area

Damage, drugs or disease to the AV node, slowing down the impulse through the AV node and down to the ventricles.

Normal Conduction

First Degree Heart Block (FHB)

Here is a rhythm that has a conduction problem in the AV node (it is more of a delay in the conduction transmission more than a block). The impulse starts off as a normal P wave, followed by a normal QRS complex, then a T wave, but if we look closely, we see that the PR interval is **not** normal, it is **greater** than 3-5 small squares (>0.20 secs).

What seems to happen is the impulse from the SA node fires off ok and there is a depolarisation through the atria Mexican Wave), but the AV node is slow to release the signal (slow action potential) as if it was a little bit forgetful. The impulse does go eventually to the ventricles (this happens on every beat). This shows up on the ECG as a **lengthened** PR interval (over 5 small squares wide). This rhythm could be caused by damage due to illness such as myocarditis (an infection of the heart muscle), drugs or disease to the AV node or is common in healthy children, athletes, footballers or other fit sports person. It is estimated that up to 2% of the human population may have First Degree Heart Block.

Although it may lead to other conduction problems, this is usually not a concern for most cardiologists especially if the patient is asymptomatic (have no symptoms). It is common to see after an MI.

	P Waves	PR Interval	QRS	T Wave	Rate	Rhythm
First Degree Heart Block	Yes	Long	Normal	Yes	Normal	Regular

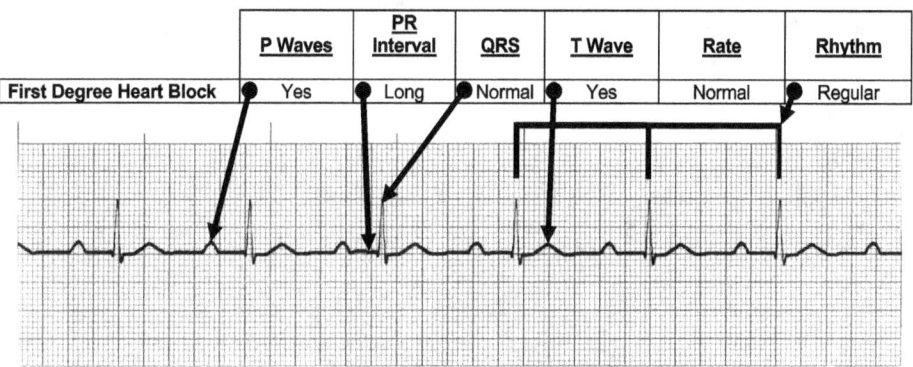

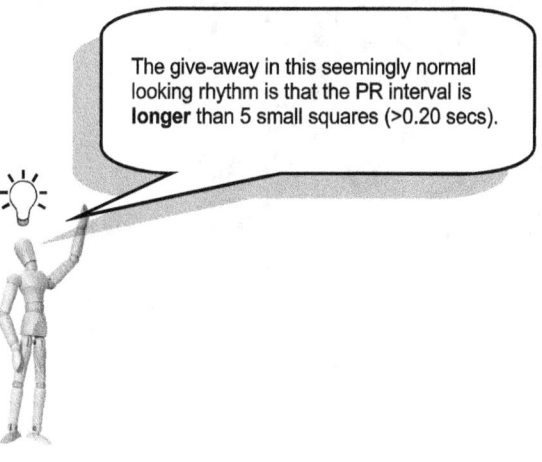

The give-away in this seemingly normal looking rhythm is that the PR interval is **longer** than 5 small squares (>0.20 secs).

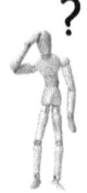

? Second Degree Heart Block Type I (Wenckebach)

	P Waves	PR Interval	QRS	T Wave	Rate	Rhythm
First Degree Heart Block	Yes	Long	Normal	Yes	Normal	Regular
Second Degree Type One	Yes	Lengthens	Normal	Not Always	Normal	Regularly Irregular
Second Degree Type Two	Yes	Sometimes	Normal	Not Always	Normal	Regular
Third Degree Heart Block	Yes	None	Wide/ Disassociated	Abnormal	Slow QRS Normal P	Regular
Bundle Branch Block	Maybe	Maybe	Wide/Notched Or Jagged	Abnormal	Normal	Regular

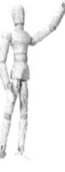

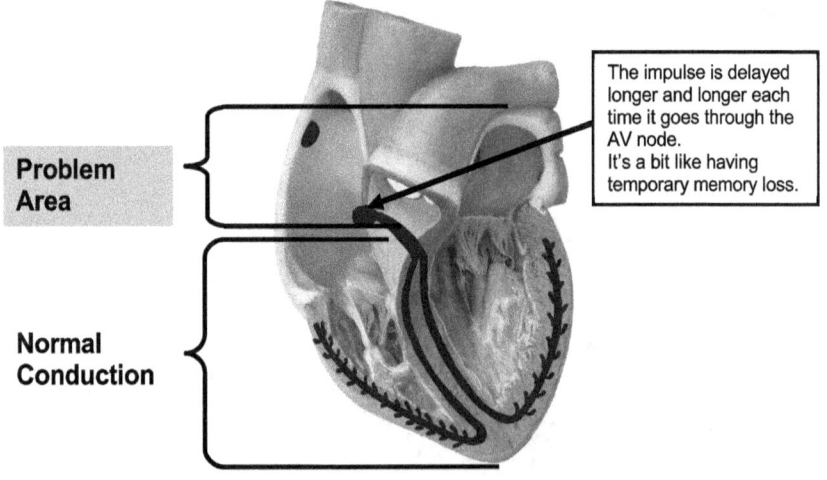

Problem Area

Normal Conduction

The impulse is delayed longer and longer each time it goes through the AV node.
It's a bit like having temporary memory loss.

Second Degree Heart Block Type I (Wenckebach)

This is another one in the not so easy category. A regularly, irregular rhythm (try saying that when your drunk never mind when you are sober! It was first described back in 1899 by Dr Karl Fredrick Wenckebach (pronounced ven-ke-bak). The impulse starts off on its normal path, SA node and atrial contraction (normal P wave) to the AV node. It is at this part that we hit a bit of a problem. The conduction through the AV node is delayed a little longer each time the impulse passes through it making the PR interval normal at first then longer and longer each beat until there is a complete block and one of the P shows up on its own with no QRS complex and, no T wave (Oh dear!) and then reverts to a normal beat (normal P wave, normal PR interval, normal QRS complex, T wave) before starting all this up again (repeat and rewind), some people analyse the rhythm backwards as "walking back" (normal, delay,delay, drop). So, the PR interval is normal, then longer and longer still, and then a P wave on its own.

It can be a pre-progression from First Degree Heart Block and in most cases It is usually determined as benign unless it is associated with an underlying heart disease or any symptomatic problems. This also can be a precursor to the next rhythm especially if the damage or blood supply is causing further decline or this rhythm. Bizarrely, this is a common rhythm found in fit athletic horses. Other causes of type I are Digitalis toxicity (from the deadly nightshade plant) or other drugs that prolong the signal in the AV node such as beta blockers and myocarditis (an infection causing the myocardium to become inflamed). It could be, though, just due to old age!

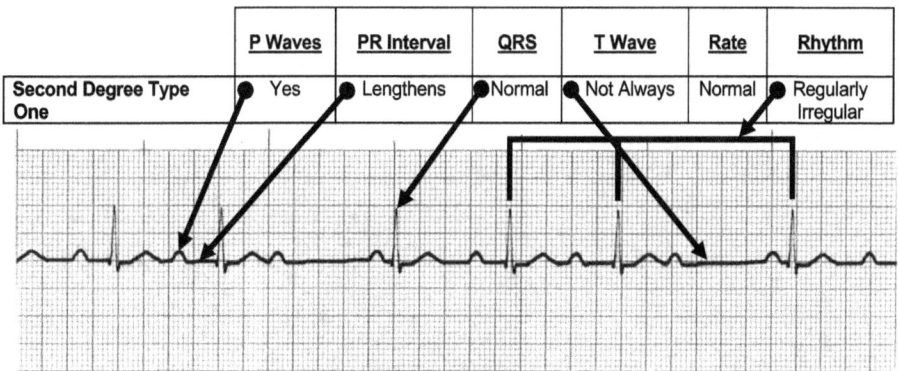

	P Waves	PR Interval	QRS	T Wave	Rate	Rhythm
Second Degree Type One	Yes	Lengthens	Normal	Not Always	Normal	Regularly Irregular

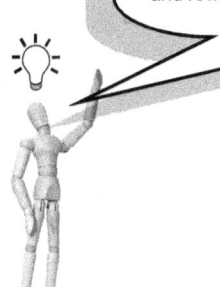

Yet another tricky little devil. The rhythm is **regularly irregular**. Find a normal beat (normal P, PR, QRS, and T) and follow the path of the P wave and the PR interval. You will see that the PR interval starts normal then, grows longer for each beat, drops a beat then goes back to normal again, and then this process starts again (repeat and rewind).

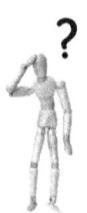

Second Degree Heart Block Type II (Mobitz)

	P Waves	PR Interval	QRS	T Wave	Rate	Rhythm
First Degree Heart Block	Yes	Long	Normal	Yes	Normal	Regular
Second Degree Type One	Yes	Lengthens	Normal	Not Always	Normal	Regularly Irregular
Second Degree Type Two	**Yes**	**Sometimes**	**Normal**	**Not Always**	**Normal**	**Regular**
Third Degree Heart Block	Yes	None	Wide/ Disassociated	Abnormal	Slow QRS Normal P	Regular
Bundle Branch Block	Maybe	Maybe	Wide/Notched Or Jagged	Abnormal	Normal	Regular

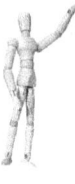

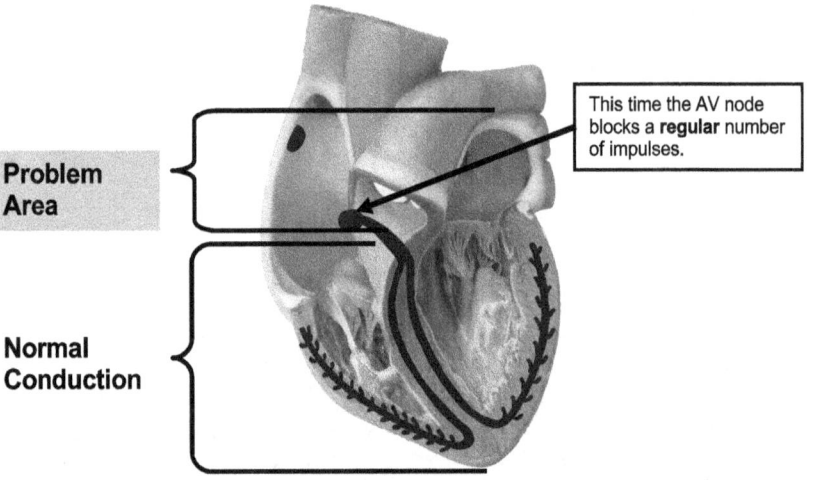

Problem Area

This time the AV node blocks a **regular** number of impulses.

Normal Conduction

Second Degree Heart Block (Mobitz Type II)

This is a regular rhythm, unlike the previous type I heart block. Not one of your easiest I am afraid, but the clue is when you see a regular set of P waves on their own. Look closely and you will see an extra normal P wave between certain QRS complexes. This is because the lesion that is causing the block is below the AV node or within the HIS bundle. It is "blocks" a regular number of impulses, i.e. every other or every three impulses (every other in this case). Because the block is below the AV node and in the HIS bundle, it can lead to 3rd Degree Heart Block. This is a constant regular block, so we can work out the severity by how many P waves there are between the QRS complexes.

Try this; if you see two P waves (counting both the one on its own **and** the normal P wave) between the QRS complexes, then this is a 2:1 (two P waves to one QRS complex) heart block. If there are three P waves between the QRS complexes, then this is a 3:1 heart block.

The difference between the two, second degree heart blocks is that the Mobitz one (Dr Woldemar Mobitz) is a **regular** rhythm while the Wenckebach (**W**-andering) is an **irregular** one.

Mobitz Type II is not as common as type one, but of course it is more serious as the disease is beyond the AV node and is lower down and at the level of the bundle branches. If seen after an anteroseptal (anterior-front) and septal (septum-middle), then the patient is at high risk of further of a very slow complete heart block (Third Degree Heart Block).

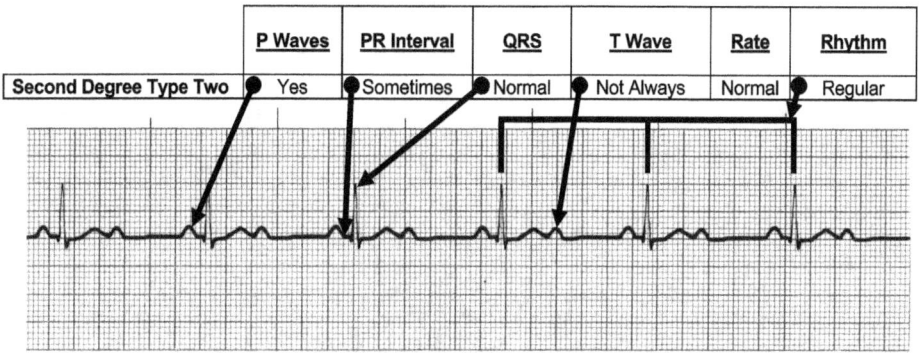

	P Waves	PR Interval	QRS	T Wave	Rate	Rhythm
Second Degree Type Two	Yes	Sometimes	Normal	Not Always	Normal	Regular

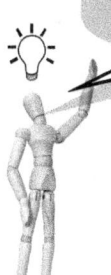

Initially it looks like a normal regular rhythm, but as you will see that in-between the QRS complexes there are lone P waves. Counting how many P waves there are between the QRS complexes gives you a constant ratio, i.e. 2:1 is two P waves between each QRS complex.

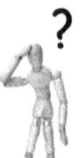

Third Degree Heart Block

	P Waves	PR Interval	QRS	T Wave	Rate	Rhythm
First Degree Heart Block	Yes	Long	Normal	Yes	Normal	Regular
Second Degree Type One	Yes	Lengthens	Normal	Not Always	Normal	Regularly Irregular
Second Degree Type Two	Yes	Sometimes	Normal	Not Always	Normal	Regular
Third Degree Heart Block	Yes	None	Wide/ Disassociated	Abnormal	Slow QRS Normal P	Regular
Bundle Branch Block	Maybe	Maybe	Wide/Notched Or Jagged	Abnormal	Normal	Regular

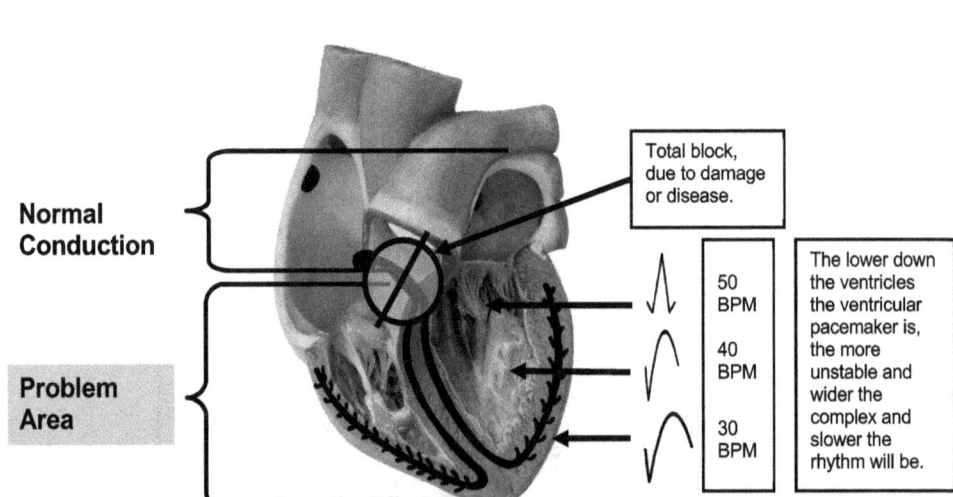

Normal Conduction

Problem Area

Total block, due to damage or disease.

50 BPM

40 BPM

30 BPM

The lower down the ventricles the ventricular pacemaker is, the more unstable and wider the complex and slower the rhythm will be.

Third degree Heart Block

This is a serious rhythm and your patient will usually feel poorly or very unwell. The QRS complexes are wide and bizarre and the initial rhythm is slow, but if you look closely, you will see that two separate rhythms are running here, the P waves and QRS are running independently of each other. It seems that the AV node has been knocked out of action, but the SA node does not know this, keeps beating away at a normal pace of about 60 - 100 BPM, and the speed can increase on exertion. The problem is that none of the impulses are getting through to the ventricles because the AV node has ceased to function anymore.

Going into survival and self-preservation mode, one of the cells in the ventricle walls decides that all is not good around him and takes control, becomes the pacemaker and beats on his own but the further down the ventricles he is, the more unstable, the slower the impulse and the wider and more bizarre the QRS will be. So up near the bundle of HIS, the QRS complex will be relatively normal and at a reasonable speed, say up about 50 BPM, but lower down in the Purkinje fibres the cell is the speed becomes about 20-30 BPM and is very wide and bizarre. At this speed, the heart may be just sustaining life, but not for long!

The atria and the ventricles are now beating at different rates to each other, the P waves running at a normal speed and the QRS complexes running at a slow speed.

The problem with this sort of speed is that the ventricles run too slow and unstable for everyday activities and are very prone to seizing up and going into Ventricular Fibrillation (see page 75) and then Asystole (see page 77). You will find the P waves and QRS complexes are both of a regular rhythm, but neither one are associated with each other. It may also be called AV dissociation in some circumstances.

Try this exercise, get a ruler or a piece of plain paper (or a pair of ECG callipers if you are lucky enough to have them, they are inexpensive and well worth it) and mark the start of one of the P waves then measure it to the start of the next P wave by sliding the marks on the paper to the next P wave and the next one and so on (look carefully as you will see that some of the P waves could be buried in the QRS complexes, see the rhythm strip below especially the 3rd complex along). You should be able to put this measurement on any part of the P wave rhythm and see that it is running as a regular rhythm. Try the same with the QRS complexes and you will see that they are both regular but work separately from each other.

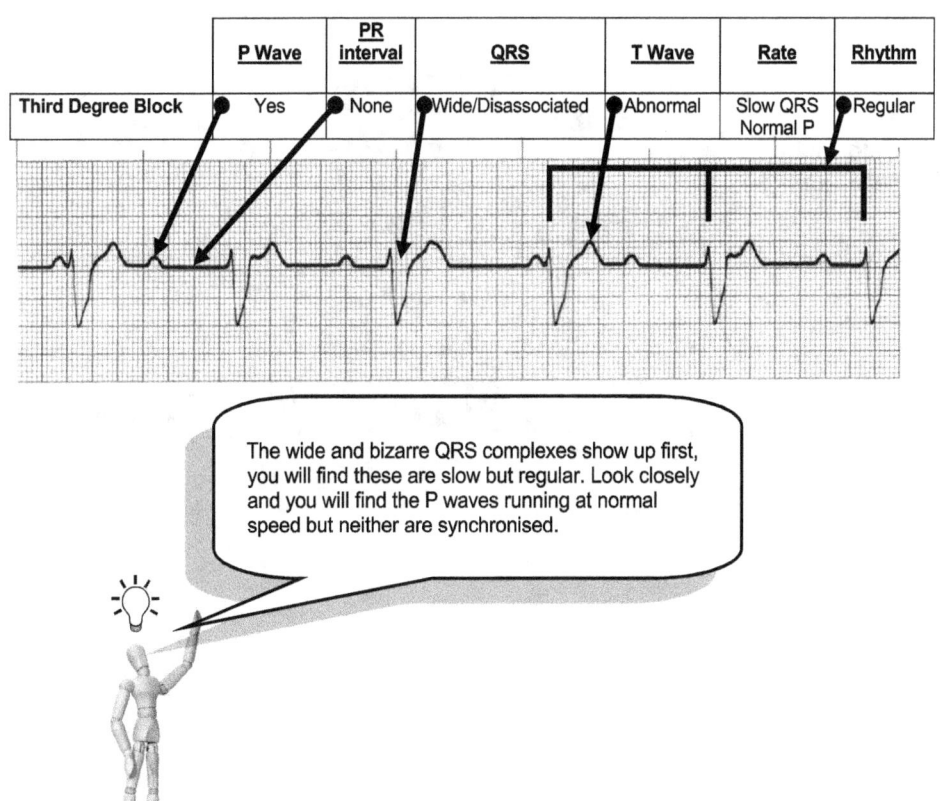

	P Wave	PR interval	QRS	T Wave	Rate	Rhythm
Third Degree Block	Yes	None	Wide/Disassociated	Abnormal	Slow QRS Normal P	Regular

The wide and bizarre QRS complexes show up first, you will find these are slow but regular. Look closely and you will find the P waves running at normal speed but neither are synchronised.

Bundle Branch Block

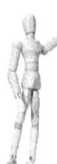

	P Waves	PR Interval	QRS	T Wave	Rate	Rhythm
First Degree Heart Block	Yes	Long	Normal	Yes	Normal	Regular
Second Degree Type One	Yes	Lengthens	Normal	Not Always	Normal	Regularly Irregular
Second Degree Type Two	Yes	Sometimes	Normal	Not Always	Normal	Regular
Third Degree Heart Block	Yes	None	Wide/ Disassociated	Abnormal	Slow QRS Normal P	Regular
Bundle Branch Block	Maybe	Maybe	Wide/Notched Or Jagged	Abnormal	Normal	Regular

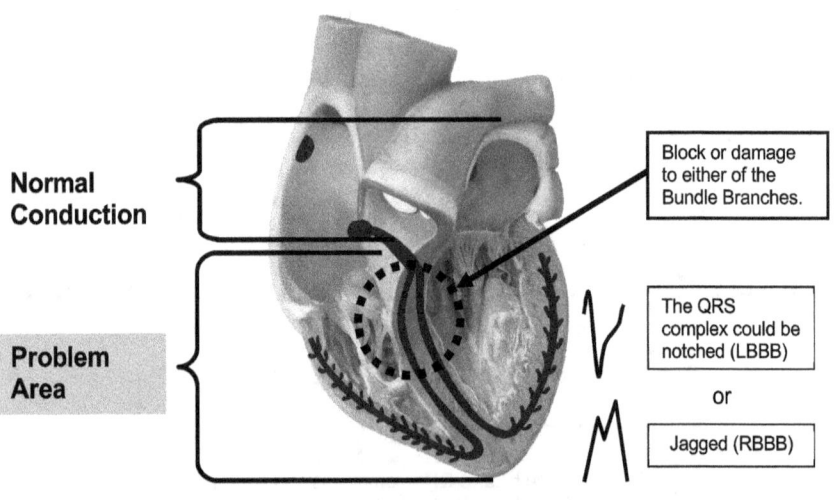

Normal Conduction

Block or damage to either of the Bundle Branches.

Problem Area

The QRS complex could be notched (LBBB)

or

Jagged (RBBB)

Bundle Branch Block (BBB)

As the name says, this is a problem with the Bundle of HIS and the bundle branches. The first thing that strikes you is that the QRS complexes are not a normal shape, they are wider than three small squares (>0.12 secs). They are not necessarily just wide or bizarre, they usually look jagged or have a notchy appearance. This is not an isolated complex the whole rhythm is like it and is very similar to the pacemaker rhythm (page 69). This is because the impulse starts off on its usual route through to the AV node; the AV node then passes the impulse down to the Bundle of HIS and it is there that it hits a block in one or both of the branches. When it reaches this block the impulse then has to find another route to get back on track, so as it is delayed in getting to the Purkinje fibres the signal is deflected causing an extra R wave or makes a notch in the complex, either way, the QRS complex is wider than three small squares. Watch that you do not get confused with the pacemaker rhythm; the giveaway if you look closely, is the pacemaker rhythm usually has obvious pacing spikes or the ECG monitor may tell you (be aware that some new pacemakers may not show pacing spikes). However, the best source of information is either the patient or one of the relatives. The block is in either the left, right or both branches, but to identify which one, you would have to take a 12 lead ECG reading. Remember though the bigger the block on one or both of the branches, the wider the QRS complexes.

The most common causes of both LBBB and RBBB are coronary artery disease, congenital abnormalities, a viarl bacterial infection such as myocarditis (inflammation of the heat muscle), hypertension (high blood pressure), a blood clot in the lung, or could be found in a small percentage of people with no heart disease at all. A LBBB can also be the result of an MI (Myocardial Infarction).

The problem with this rhythm is it is very difficult to tell if there is a severe heart problem underneath a LBBB draws a "curtain or masking effect" over the whole rhythm and obscures anything sinister that might be going on. So it is best that we say this is a very serious rhythm as we don't know what could be **really** lurking in there. If it is a RBBB then it is possible to diagnose an MI, as the left ventricle has not been affected. So of the two, the most critical and more life-threatening is the LBBB as it compromises the main heart pumping chamber which makes it pump out of sync (Due to the delay, the right ventricle is activated first and then finally to the left). Anything that compromises or weakens the left ventricle is critical.

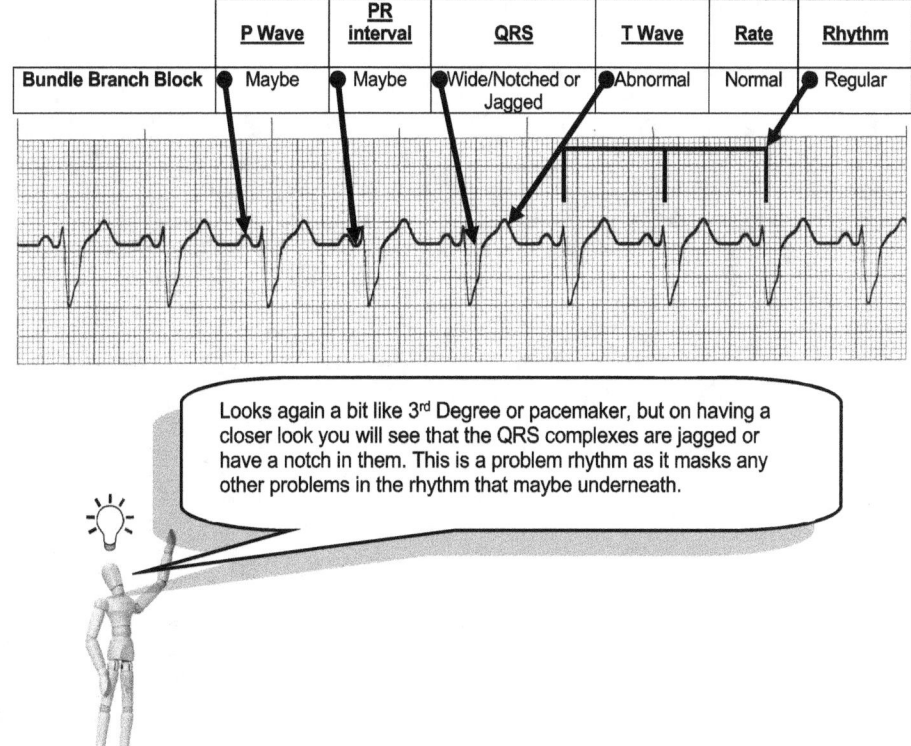

	P Wave	PR interval	QRS	T Wave	Rate	Rhythm
Bundle Branch Block	Maybe	Maybe	Wide/Notched or Jagged	Abnormal	Normal	Regular

Looks again a bit like 3rd Degree or pacemaker, but on having a closer look you will see that the QRS complexes are jagged or have a notch in them. This is a problem rhythm as it masks any other problems in the rhythm that maybe underneath.

Just to confuse matters

Just a little section to upset the applecart a little. You may find that when you look at a rhythm, there is more than one problem with the rhythm at that time. For example, you may see an Atrial Fibrillation rhythm that has Ventricular Ectopics in amongst it. The thing to do is, find out what the underlying rhythm is first then work out what the other problem or problems are. So from below, we would take the Atrial Fibrillation rhythm first with the Ventricular Ectopic second. Another may be 1st Degree Heart Block with Atrial Ectopics, the 1st Degree Block is the underlying rhythm and should be noted first and the Atrial Ectopics are the other considerations.

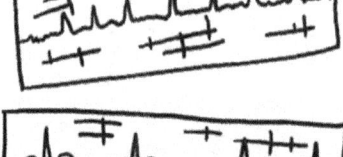

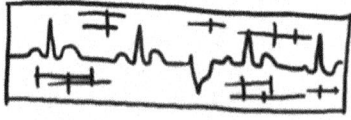

So remember, <u>**UNDERLYING RHYTHM FIRST**</u>.

Atrial Fibrillation (initial rhythm)

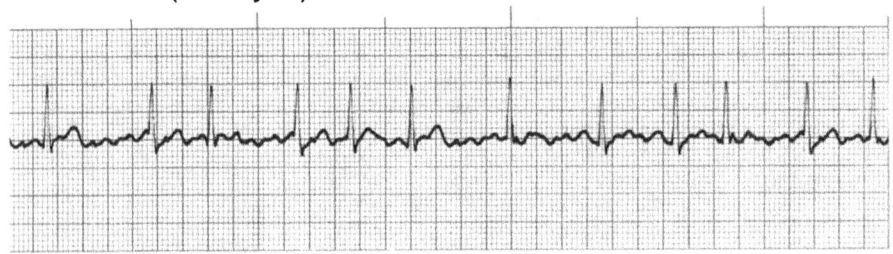

Premature Ventricular Contractions (secondary problem)

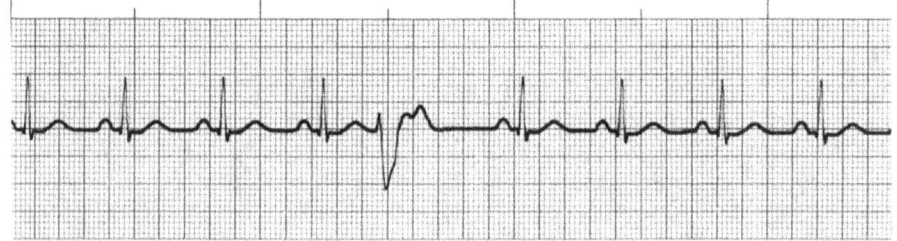

I Did It My Way

One of the hardest parts of reading the ECG is a quick recognition (don't we know it!!).
Is it an Atrial or ventricular problem? One-way I have found helps (remember this does not work for all rhythms but nearly all) is to look quickly at the complex as a whole. If the QRS is normal, then it is usually an **Atrial** problem. If the QRS is wide and bizarre, then it is usually a **Ventricular** problem.
Try this as an exercise, quickly look at this rhythm below and quickly determine if the problem is an Atrial or Ventricular one, it should only take you a few seconds to work it out.

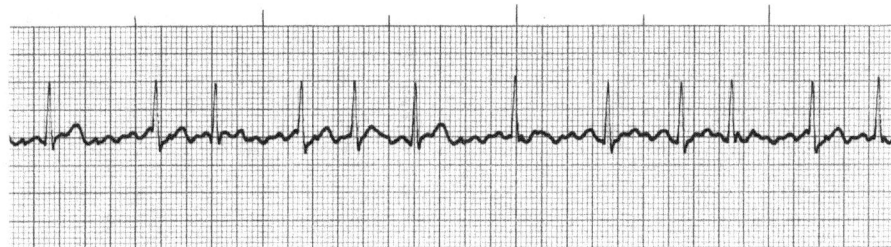

The QRS complexes are normal, so it is an **Atrial** problem. Let's see if we can work out using the powers of deduction what rhythm it is.
So what strikes you next is the rate and you will see that it is fast. There is an average of 2-3 large squares between the R waves of the QRS complexes, which gives us an approx. speed of 120 BPM. It is **fast**; so then you can deduct all those that have a slow or normal heart rate, which leaves us with 7 rhythms.

	P Waves	PR Interval	QRS	T Wave	Rate	Rhythm
Sinus Rhythm	Yes	Normal	Normal	Yes	Normal 60-100	Regular
Sinus Tachycardia	Yes	Normal	Normal	Yes	Fast 100-120	Regular
Sinus Bradycardia	Yes	Normal	Normal	Yes	Slow <60	Regular
Sinus Arrhythmia	Yes	Normal	Normal	Yes	Normal	Irregular
Atrial Tachycardia	Don't know	No	Normal	Don't know	Fast 120-140	Regular
SVT	Don't know	No	Normal	Don't know	Fast 140+	Regular
Atrial Fibrillation	F Waves	Don't know	Normal	Don't know	Fast 120+	Irregular
Atrial Flutter	Sawtoothed	Don't know	Normal	Don't know	Normal or Fast	Regular
Atrial Ectopic (Sinus)	Yes	Yes	Normal	Yes	Any	Irregular
Junctional Ectopic	No	No	Normal	Yes	Any	Irregular
First Degree Heart Block	Yes	Long	Normal	Yes	Normal	Regular
Second Degree Type One	Yes	Lengthens	Normal	Not Always	Normal	Regularly Irregular
Second Degree Type Two	Yes	Sometimes	Normal	Not Always	Normal	Regular

The next thing that we look for is if the rhythm is regular of irregular. We see that it is in fact **irregular**, so what we do is to remove all the rhythms with regular heartbeats.

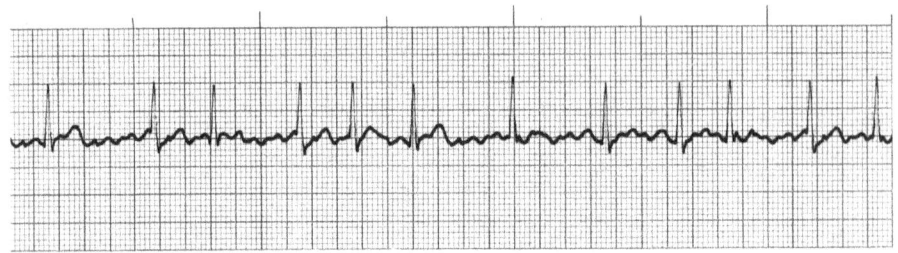

	P Waves	PR Interval	QRS	T Wave	Rate	Rhythm
~~Sinus Rhythm~~	~~Yes~~	~~Normal~~	~~Normal~~	~~Yes~~	~~Normal 60-100~~	~~Regular~~
~~Sinus Tachycardia~~	~~Yes~~	~~Normal~~	~~Normal~~	~~Yes~~	~~Fast 100-120~~	~~Regular~~
~~Sinus Bradycardia~~	~~Yes~~	~~Normal~~	~~Normal~~	~~Yes~~	~~Slow <60~~	~~Regular~~
Sinus Arrhythmia	Yes	Normal	Normal	Yes	Normal	Irregular
~~Atrial Tachycardia~~	~~Don't know~~	~~No~~	~~Normal~~	~~Don't know~~	~~Fast 120-140~~	~~Regular~~
~~SVT~~	~~Don't know~~	~~No~~	~~Normal~~	~~Don't know~~	~~Fast 140+~~	~~Regular~~
Atrial Fibrillation	F Waves	Don't know	Normal	Don't know	Fast 120+	Irregular
~~Atrial Flutter~~	Sawtoothed	~~Don't know~~	Normal	Don't know	Normal or Fast	Regular
Atrial Ectopic (Sinus)	Yes	Yes	Normal	Yes	Any	Irregular
Junctional Ectopic	No	No	Normal	Yes	Any	Irregular
~~First Degree Heart Block~~	~~Yes~~	~~Long~~	~~Normal~~	~~Yes~~	~~Normal~~	~~Regular~~
~~Second Degree Type One~~	~~Yes~~	~~Lengthens~~	~~Normal~~	~~Not Always~~	~~Normal~~	~~Regularly Irregular~~
~~Second Degree Type Two~~	~~Yes~~	~~Sometimes~~	~~Normal~~	~~Not Always~~	~~Normal~~	~~Regular~~

We are now left with just three rhythms. To be absolutely sure, check to see if there are any normal P waves. On this rhythm, we are not sure if they **are** P waves, but there is something there, so the first thing to do is rule out any muscle tremor or interference. That done, they must be F Waves. Let's now knock off the junctional ectopics because they do not have **normal** P waves anyway. We are now left with **two.**

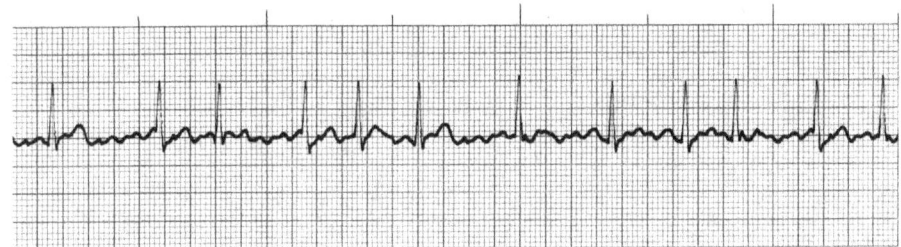

	P Waves	PR Interval	QRS	T Wave	Rate	Rhythm
Sinus Rhythm	Yes	Normal	Normal	Yes	Normal 60-100	Regular
Sinus Tachycardia	Yes	Normal	Normal	Yes	Fast 100-120	Regular
Sinus Bradycardia	Yes	Normal	Normal	Yes	Slow <60	Regular
Sinus Arrhythmia	Yes	Normal	Normal	Yes	Normal	Irregular
Atrial Tachycardia	Don't know	No	Normal	Don't know	Fast 120-140	Regular
SVT	Don't know	No	Normal	Don't know	Fast 140+	Regular
Atrial Fibrillation	F Waves	Don't know	Normal	Don't know	Fast 120+	Irregular
Atrial Flutter	Sawtoothed	Don't know	Normal	Don't know	Normal or Fast	Regular
Atrial Ectopic (Sinus)	Yes	Yes	Normal	Yes	Any	Irregular
Junctional Ectopic	No	No	Normal	Yes	Any	Irregular
First Degree Heart Block	Yes	Long	Normal	Yes	Normal	Regular
Second Degree Type One	Yes	Lengthens	Normal	Not Always	Normal	Regularly Irregular
Second Degree Type Two	Yes	Sometimes	Normal	Not Always	Normal	Regular

Right then, let's check out the PR interval, well we are still not sure about the normal P waves, they look like F waves. So if this is the case we can get rid of the Sinus Atrial Ectopics as they have a normal PR interval and that leaves us with only on rhythm left that is **Atrial Fibrillation.** Phew!
Do you get it yet?

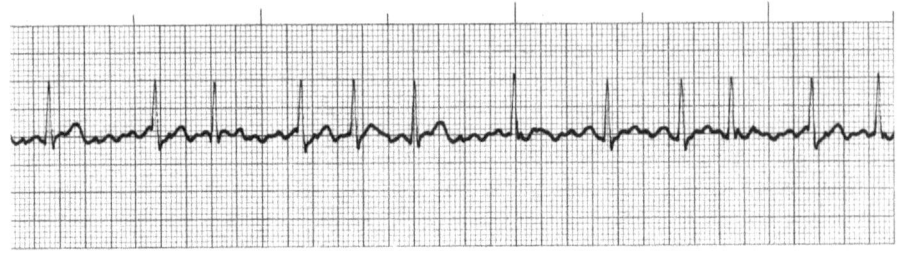

	P Waves	PR Interval	QRS	T Wave	Rate	Rhythm
Sinus Rhythm	Yes	Normal	Normal	Yes	Normal 60-100	Regular
Sinus Tachycardia	Yes	Normal	Normal	Yes	Fast 100-120	Regular
Sinus Bradycardia	Yes	Normal	Normal	Yes	Slow <60	Regular
Sinus Arrhythmia	Yes	Normal	Normal	Yes	Normal	Irregular
Atrial Tachycardia	Don't know	No	Normal	Don't know	Fast 120-140	Regular
SVT	Don't know	No	Normal	Don't know	Fast 140+	Regular
Atrial Fibrillation	F Waves	Don't know	Normal	Don't know	Fast 120+	Irregular
Atrial Flutter	Sawtoothed	Don't know	Normal	Don't know	Normal or Fast	Regular
Atrial Ectopic (Sinus)	Yes	Yes	Normal	Yes	Any	Irregular
Junctional Ectopic	No	No	Normal	Yes	Any	Irregular
First Degree Heart Block	Yes	Long	Normal	Yes	Normal	Regular
Second Degree Type One	Yes	Lengthens	Normal	Not Always	Normal	Regularly Irregular
Second Degree Type Two	Yes	Sometimes	Normal	Not Always	Normal	Regular

Let's try another. Look at the overall rhythm below; are the QRS normal or wide and bizarre?

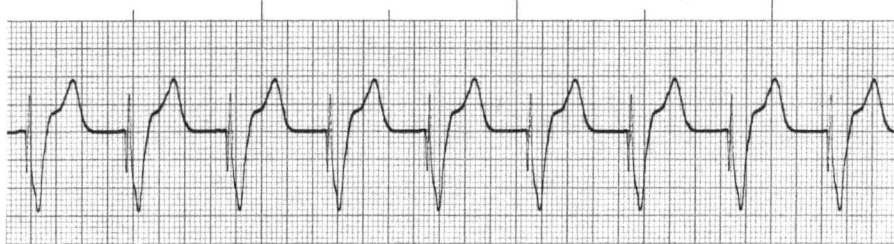

The QRS complexes are **Wide and Bizarre** so we find that this is a **Ventricular** problem so there is no need for the atrial rhythm list. The rate you find is **normal** as the average large squares between the R waves in the QRS complexes are 4 which is about 70 BPM, so we can rule out all the fast and slow rhythms.

	P Wave	PR Interval	QRS	T Wave	Rate	Rhythm
Ventricular Ectopic	No	None	Wide/Bizarre	Abnormal	Normal	Irregular
R on T Ectopic	No	None	Wide/Bizarre	Abnormal	Normal	Irregular
Bigeminal Ectopic	No	None	Wide/Bizarre	Abnormal	Slow	Regular
Third Degree Block	Yes	None	Wide/Disassociated	Abnormal	Slow QRS Normal P	Regular
Pacemaker	Maybe	Maybe	Wide/Bizarre With Pacing Spikes	Abnormal	Normal	Regular
Ventricular Tachycardia	Maybe	None	Wide	No	Very Fast	Regular
Ventricular Fibrillation	Don't know	None	Disorganised	Don't know	Very Fast	Irregular
Asystole	No	None	None	No	None	None
Bundle Branch Block	Maybe	Maybe	Wide/Notched or Jagged	Abnormal	Normal	Regular

That leaves us with only **four** rhythms now, so let's look a bit deeper and see if we can narrow them down even further. Is the rhythm regular? Yes, it is. Right, get rid of the irregular ones.

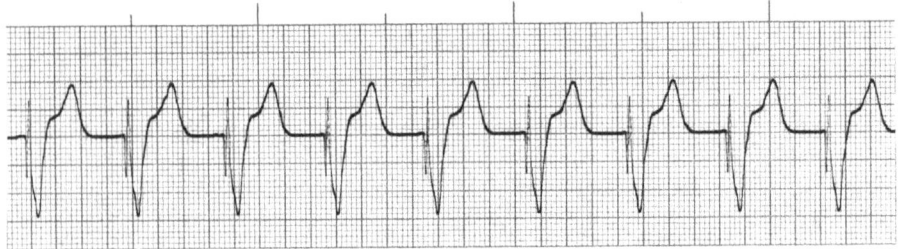

	P Wave	PR Interval	QRS	T Wave	Rate	Rhythm
~~Ventricular Ectopic~~	~~No~~	~~None~~	~~Wide/Bizarre~~	~~Abnormal~~	~~Normal~~	~~Irregular~~
~~R on T Ectopic~~	~~No~~	~~None~~	~~Wide/Bizarre~~	~~Abnormal~~	~~Normal~~	~~Irregular~~
~~Bigeminal Ectopic~~	~~No~~	~~None~~	~~Wide/Bizarre~~	~~Abnormal~~	~~Slow~~	~~Regular~~
~~Third Degree Block~~	~~Yes~~	~~None~~	~~Wide/Disassociated~~	~~Abnormal~~	~~Slow QRS Normal P~~	~~Regular~~
Pacemaker	Maybe	Maybe	Wide/Bizarre With Pacing Spikes	Abnormal	Normal	Regular
~~Ventricular Tachycardia~~	~~Maybe~~	~~None~~	~~Wide~~	~~No~~	~~Very Fast~~	~~Regular~~
~~Ventricular Fibrillation~~	~~Don't know~~	~~None~~	~~Disorganised~~	~~Don't know~~	~~Very Fast~~	~~Irregular~~
~~Asystole~~	~~No~~	~~None~~	~~None~~	~~No~~	~~None~~	~~None~~
Bundle Branch Block	Maybe	Maybe	Wide/Notched or Jagged	Abnormal	Normal	Regular

We are now left with just **two**. Just to be sure, the obvious part of this rhythm is that the QRS complexes have **Pacing Spikes** at the start. So there you go a **Pacemaker Rhythm**. Well Done!

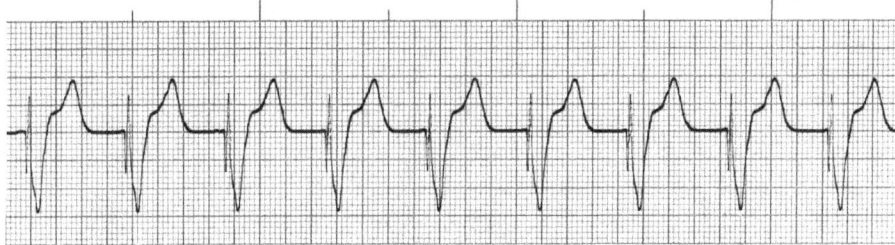

	P Wave	PR Interval	QRS	T Wave	Rate	Rhythm
Ventricular Ectopic	No	None	Wide/Bizarre	Abnormal	Normal	Irregular
R on T Ectopic	No	None	Wide/Bizarre	Abnormal	Normal	Irregular
Bigeminal Ectopic	No	None	Wide/Bizarre	Abnormal	Slow	Regular
Third Degree Block	Yes	None	Wide/Disassociated	Abnormal	Slow QRS Normal P	Regular
Pacemaker	Maybe	Maybe	Wide/Bizarre With Pacing Spikes	Abnormal	Normal	Regular
Ventricular Tachycardia	Maybe	None	Wide	No	Very Fast	Regular
Ventricular Fibrillation	Don't know	None	Disorganised	No	Very Fast	Irregular
Asystole	No	None	None	None	None	None
Bundle Branch Block	Maybe	Maybe	Wide/Notched or Jagged	Abnormal	Normal	Regular

A Testing Time

Now for the dreaded moment, the small test to see how much has sunk in! Just have a go to see how you get on, don't just recognise the rhythms try and work out what is happening to each one. The answers are on page 102, so you can cheat if you want but just remember, the only person that you are cheating on is yourself! If it helps, use the charts on page 108 for reference, but please give it an honest go, you might be surprised how much you have learnt.

Let's start you off with a nice easy one.

1.

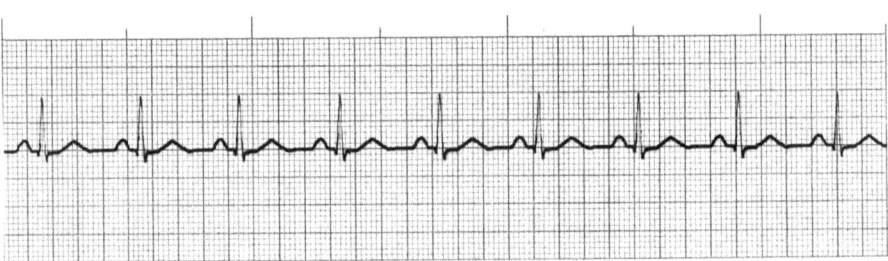

2.

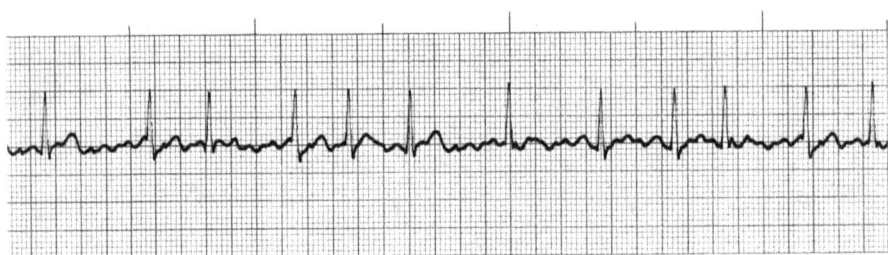

3.

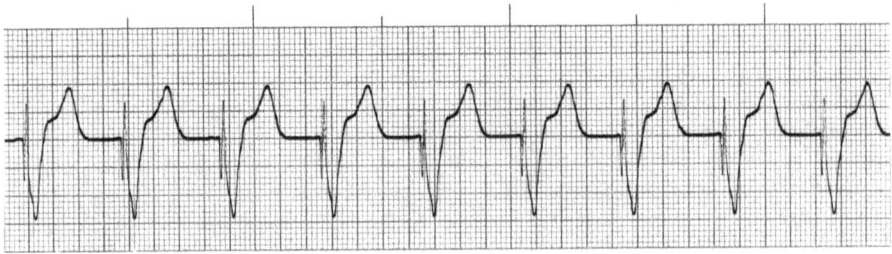

4.

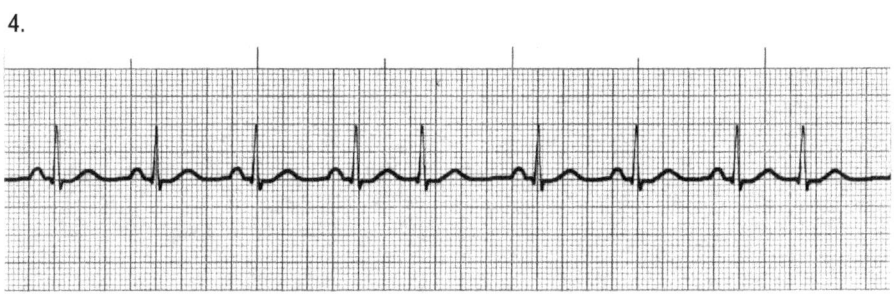

5.

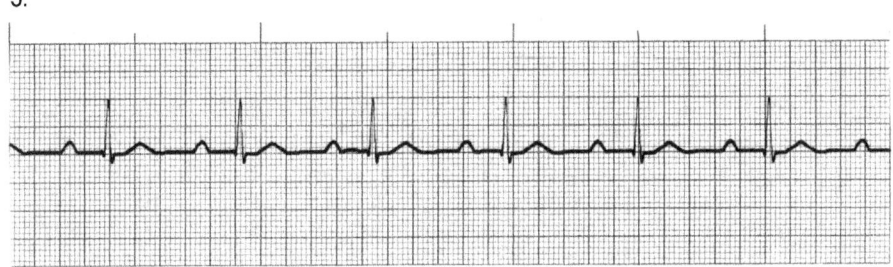

6.

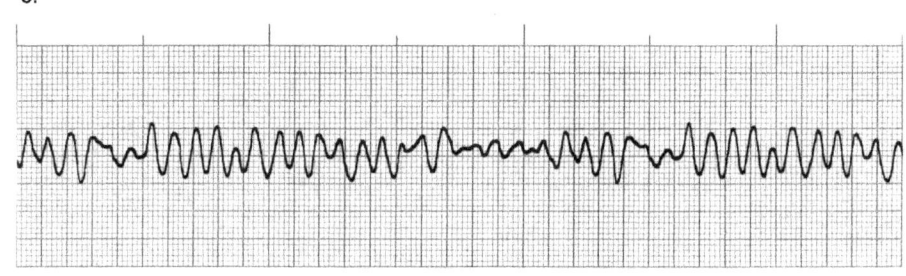

7.

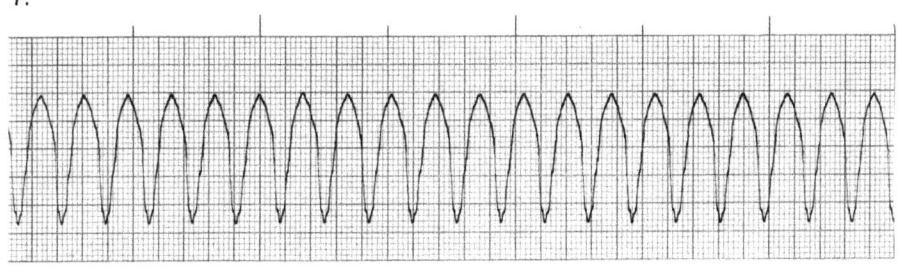

8.

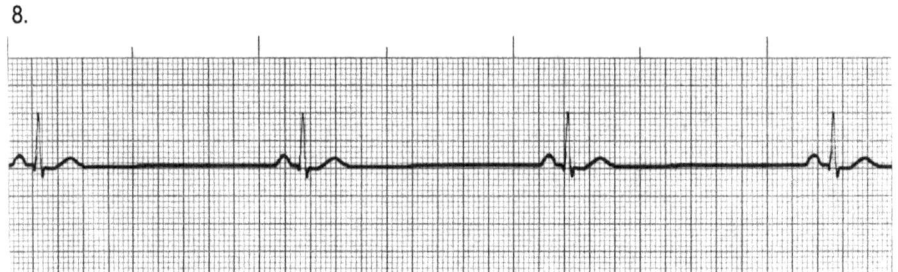

9.

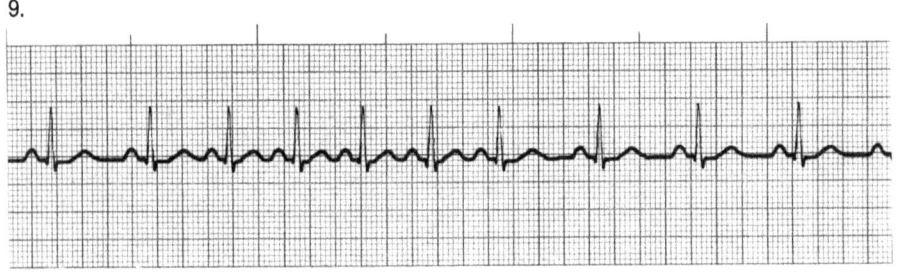

Answers

Well here are the answers to the test, I hope you didn't cheat! We started with an easy one:

1.   This is **Sinus Rhythm**. A quick glance tells us that this is an **Atrial** rhythm, because the QRS complexes are normal not wide and bizarre. There is a P wave followed by a QRS then a T wave. The rate is between 60 – 100 BPM and the rhythm is **regular**, therefore this cannot be anything else other than **Normal Sinus Rhythm.**
2.   **Atrial Fibrillation** is our next one. Again an **Atrial** problem, the main thing that strikes you is the rhythm being **irregular**, and it is difficult to see if there are P or T waves in-between the QRS complexes. After ruling out muscle tremor and atrial flutter (atrial flutter is a **regular** rhythm), you are left with **Atrial Fibrillation.**
3.   This is a **Pacemaker** rhythm. Can be confused with third degree heart block, but the **pacing spikes** give the game away.
4.   These are **Junctional Ectopics.** If you look at the rhythm it appears to be normal apart from the odd glitch. These extra beats also appear normal at first but if you look closely enough you will see that they have **no P** waves.
5.   Here we have **First-degree heart block**. Again a seemingly normal rhythm but the **PR** interval is longer than **5 small squares**, which tells us that there is a problem with the AV node.
6.   This is a big bad Oh dear! rhythm, it is **Ventricular Fibrillation**. This one you will find is obvious, but the first thing you must do is, make sure that this is not interference, or a loose lead or electrode problem. The other clue to this is that the patient will be unconscious and have no pulse.
7.   Another one of the Oh dear! section, **Ventricular Tachycardia**. Distinctive by its "**Deckchair looking**" wide and bizarre complexes, and its regularity. If you look into the complexes you might just see some **P waves** cropping up now and again.
8.   A nice and easy one for you now, **Sinus Bradycardia**. A nice straightforward rhythm, with everything in place except for the fact that it is much **too slow** to be Normal Sinus Rhythm.
9.   And for the final one we have **Sinus Arrhythmia**, looks like Normal Sinus Rhythm but it seems that every so often the rhythm **speeds up then returns to normal**. For this one check your patients breathing pattern and if it speeds up when they breathe in and return to normal when they breathe out then there is your answer!

Glossary (Or What Does That Word Mean Again!)

- **Action Potential** - The change in electrical potential associated with the passage of an impulse along the membrane of a muscle cell or nerve cell.
- **AED** - Automated External Defibrillator. A small battery operated portable device that is used in cardiac arrest and recognises ventricular fibrillation and ventricular tachycardia and delivers a controlled electrical discharge to enable the heart's natural pacemaker to regain natural control.
- **Anterior** - Nearer the front of the body. The opposite of posterior
- **Asymptomatic** - Without symptoms.
- **Atria** - Roman for an inner courtyard open to the sky, or in medical terms the upper chambers of the heart that receives blood from the veins.
- **Atrioventricular (AV)** - Meaning both atriums and ventricles.
- **Arrhythmia** - An abnormal pulse rhythm due to disturbance of the heart's pacemaker.
- **Asymptomatic** - Without symptoms.
- **Asystole** (pronounced **ay-sis-tollee**) - The total absence of any electrical activity in the heart. Cardiac Arrest.
- **Bachmann Bundle** - A division of the anterior atrial intermodal tract that continues across into the left atrium providing a connection between the two atrial chambers.
- **Baseline** - An imaginary horizontal line drawn straight through an ECG rhythm where the P, QRS and T waves should start and finish.
- **Bradycardia** - An abnormally slow pulse, <60 BPM (Beats Per Minute).
- **Bluetooth**-is both a Danish Viking Danish King Harald king Blåtand and a wireless technology standard for exchanging data over short distances on electronic devices.
- **Brugada Syndrome** - A genetic cardiac disease that involves the sodium ion channel and produces Electrocardiograph abnormalities.
- **Bundle of HIS** (pronounced **Hiss**) - Just below the Atrioventricular (AV) node named after a German chap named HIS, which divides into two, the left and right branches called the bundle branches.
- **Bundle Branches** - Lead off the bundle of HIS and divide into the left and right branches. The left branch feeds the left side of the heart, as the right bundle branch feeds the right hand side.
- **BPM** - Beats Per Minute
- **Bigeminy** (pronounced **buy-gem-inee**) - Every other beat
- **Cardiac Arrest** - An unconscious person with no pulse and is not breathing. They are clinically dead.
- **Cardioversion** - Is a medical procedure by which an abnormally fast heart rate (tachycardia) or cardiac arrhythmia is converted to a normal rhythm, using electricity or drugs.
- **Complex** - Small parts made into a big part e.g. the QRS complex is made up of the Q wave, the R and the S wave and are linked to form one complex i.e. the QRS complex.
- **Conduction** - Nothing to do with orchestras but the passing of an electrical current through something.
- **Defibrillator** - An electronic device capable of delivering short bursts of high voltage current to stun the heart and possibly restore Ventricular Fibrillation or pulseless Ventricular Tachycardia to a normal heart rhythm.
- **Ectopic** - An extra heartbeat, sometimes known as an extrasystole (pronounced **extra-sis-tollee**)
- **ECG** - Electro Cardio Graph, a machine used to observe the electrical activity of the heart picked up from the surface of the skin by attaching electrodes to the surface if the skin.
- **Einthoven's Triangle** - Arranging the ECG leads on a patient to form a triangle. Named after a gentleman called Willem Einthoven!
- **Electrode** - A sticky pad with a metal conductor inserted, which picks up the electrical impulse when stuck to the surface of the skin and attached by leads to an ECG monitor.
- **Endocardium** - This is the innermost layer of tissue that lines the chambers of the heart.
- **Epicardium** - This is the outer layer of the heart.
- **Fibrosis** - The formation of excess fibrous connective tissue in an organ or tissue (effectively "scarring" of tissue).
- **Foci** - The centre of interest or activity.
- **Fibrillation** - Fine rapid twitching of the heart's muscle fibres.
- **Flatline** - A flat straight line shown on an ECG monitor, slang for the rhythm Asystole

- **Flutter** - Rapid regular twitching of heart muscle
- **F Waves** - Indefinable electrical activity between the QRS complexes in a rhythm (after ruling out any
- interference or muscle tremor). If you are unsure of its identity, then it is called an F wave.
- **Heart Block** - Damage or disease in the conduction system causing a block in the normal travels of a heart impulse.
- **Holter** - A portable ambulatory electrocardiography device that continuously monitors cardiac or brain activities for 24 hours up to 2 weeks in duration.
- **Idiopathic** - Greek for "a disease of its own kind". Of unknown cause.
- **Impulse** - The discharge of electrical energy.
- **Inferior** - Situated below or directly downwards. Closer to the feet than another. The lower surface of a structure.
- **Ions** - These are electrically charged particles which are formed when atoms lose or gain electrons (electrons are the negatively charged particles of an atom).
- **Macroreentry Circuit** - A current that circles around a large normal or abnormal structure.
- **Microreentry Circuit** - Involving a small circuit such as one that is within the atrioventricular or in the Purkinje fibres.
- **Millivolts** - One thousandth of a volt.
- **Myocardium (my-o-car-di-um)** -The muscular tissue of the heart (the middle bit).
- **Node** - A group of specialised nerve cells capable of producing an electrical impulse.
- **Pacemaker** - Something that takes control. As in the case of the heart, it has a natural pacemaker which is the Sino Atrial (SA) node placed high up the wall of the right Atria. The other type is a manmade electrical device which is implanted into the chest wall and takes control of the heart beats in a damaged or diseased heart.
- **Purkinje (pronounced-purr-kin-gee) Fibres** - Spidery type nerves imbedded into the heart muscle in the Ventricles and are the end of the hearts impulse, and they make the muscles in the ventricles contract causing the blood to be pumped out to the body's systems.
- **Re-entry** - The action or process of re-entering something. The return of the same impulse into an area of the heart muscle that it has recently activated but that is now no longer refractory.
- **Refractory** - Not responding to stimulus.
- **Repolarising** - Returning the membrane potential back to its resting membrane potential (recharging to its ready status).
- **SADS** - Sudden Arrhythmic Death Syndrome.
- **Septum** - A wall of muscle dividing the two ventricles.
- **Sinus**-No not a Roman Emperor, but anything originating from the Sino Atrial (SA) node.
- **Sino Atrial (SA) Node**-This is the heart's natural pacemaker and where all the impulses start from.
- **Sodium-potassium Pump** - A membrane-bound transporter found in nearly all mammalian cells that transports potassium ions into the cytoplasm from the extracellular fluid while simultaneously transporting sodium ions out of the cytoplasm to the extracellular fluid.
- **Supra Ventricular Tachycardia (SVT)** - Supra means above, and tachycardia means as below, a fast rate of >100 BPM, so SVT is a fast rhythm above the heart's ventricles.
- **Tachycardia** - A fast heart rate of >100 Beats Per Minute.
- **Torsade-De-Pointes** - French for "twisting on spikes". It is a polymorphic (taking on different forms) ventricular tachycardia that usually self terminates. It is also a ballet movement.
- **Vena Cave** - The large veins that return the deoxygenated blood to the heart.
- **Ventricles** - It means a small pouch or cavity. Medically it means the two bottom pumping chambers of the heart.
- **Wolfe Parkinson White Syndrome** - This is a disorder of the heart's electrical system with an abnormal accessory pathway. Commonly known as a pre-excitation syndrome

Index

You might find these of use as a quick reference. Please feel free to cut them out.

Atrial Rhythms

	P Waves	PR Interval	QRS	T Wave	Rate	Rhythm
Sinus Rhythm	Yes	Normal	Normal	Yes	Normal 60-100	Regular
Sinus Tachycardia	Yes	Normal	Normal	Yes	Fast 100-120	Regular
Sinus Bradycardia	Yes	Normal	Normal	Yes	Slow <60	Regular
Sinus Arrhythmia	Yes	Normal	Normal	Yes	Normal	Irregular
Atrial Tachycardia	Don't know	No	Normal	Don't know	Fast 120-140	Regular
SVT	Don't know	No	Normal	Don't know	Fast 140+	Regular
Atrial Fibrillation	F Waves	Don't know	Normal	Don't know	Fast 120+	Irregular
Atrial Flutter	Sawtoothed	Don't know	Normal	Don't know	Normal or Fast	Regular
Atrial Ectopic (Sinus)	Yes	Yes	Normal	Yes	Any	Irregular
Junctional Ectopic	No	No	Normal	Yes	Any	Irregular
First Degree Heart Block	Yes	Long	Normal	Yes	Normal	Regular
Second Degree Type One	Yes	Lengthens	Normal	Not Always	Normal	Regularly Irregular
Second Degree Type Two	Yes	Sometimes	Normal	Not Always	Normal	Regular

Ventricular Rhythms

	P Wave	PR Interval	QRS	T Wave	Rate	Rhythm
Ventricular Ectopic	No	None	Wide/Bizarre	Abnormal	Normal	Irregular
R on T Ectopic	No	None	Wide/Bizarre	Abnormal	Normal	Irregular
Bigeminal Ectopic	No	None	Wide/Bizarre	Abnormal	Slow	Regular
Third Degree Block	Yes	None	Wide/Disassociated	Abnormal	Slow QRS Normal P	Regular
Pacemaker	Maybe	Maybe	Wide/Bizarre with pacing spikes	Abnormal	Normal	Regular
Ventricular Tachycardia	Maybe	None	Wide	No	Very Fast	Regular
Ventricular Fibrillation	Don't know	None	Disorganised	Don't know	Very Fast	Irregular
Asystole	No	None	None	No	None	None
Bundle Branch Block	Maybe	Maybe	Wide/Notched or Jagged	Abnormal	Normal	Regular

Notes Page — (Just somewhere to scribble what you think)